SHARED DECISION MAKING AND SERIOUS MENTAL ILLNESS

SHARED DECISION MAKING AND SERIOUS MENTAL ILLNESS

EDITED BY
PATRICK W. CORRIGAN

AMERICAN PSYCHOLOGICAL ASSOCIATION

Published by
American Psychological Association
750 First Street, NE
Washington, DC 20002
https://www.apa.org

Order Department
https://www.apa.org/pubs/books
order@apa.org

Typeset in Charter and Interstate by Circle Graphics, Inc., Reisterstown, MD

Printer: Gasch Printing, Odenton, MD
Cover Designer: Gwen J. Grafft, Minneapolis, MN

Library of Congress Cataloging-in-Publication Data

CIP data has been applied for. Library of Congress Cataloging in Publication Control Number: 2025018051.

ISBN 9781433843983 (paperback)
ISBN 9781433843990 (epub)
ISBN 9781433849923 (pdf)

https://doi.org/10.1037/0000478-000

Printed in the United States of America

10 9 8 7 6 5 4 3 2 1

To Georgeen Carson, my life partner and inspiration,
regardless of what life throws at us.

Contents

Contributors

Sarah E. Coates, BS, Illinois Institute of Technology, Chicago, IL, United States

Deborah A. Cohen, PhD, Dell Medical School, Steve Hicks School of Social Work, The University of Texas at Austin, Austin, TX, United States

Patrick W. Corrigan, PsyD, Illinois Institute of Technology, Chicago, IL, United States

Rebecca P. Johnson, MA, Texas Institute for Excellence in Mental Health, Steve Hicks School of Social Work, The University of Texas at Austin, Austin, TX, United States

Vardha Kharbanda, MA, Illinois Institute of Technology, Chicago, IL, United States

Vanessa V. Klodnick, PhD, Texas Institute for Excellence in Mental Health, Steve Hicks School of Social Work, The University of Texas at Austin, Austin, TX, United States

Brianne LaPelusa, MFA, Texas Institute for Excellence in Mental Health, Steve Hicks School of Social Work, The University of Texas at Austin, Austin, TX, United States

Abby Mayhue, BA, DePaul University, Chicago, IL; Texas Institute for Excellence in Mental Health, Steve Hicks School of Social Work, The University of Texas at Austin, Austin, TX, United States

Rachel Parson, BA, Illinois Institute of Technology, Chicago, IL, United States

Lindsay Sheehan, PhD, Illinois Institute of Technology, Chicago, IL, United States

Virginia Spicknall, MS, Illinois Institute of Technology, Chicago, IL, United States

Karyn Bolden Stovall, MSW, MA, Chicago State University, Chicago, IL, United States

Sai Snigdha Talluri, PhD, Yale School of Medicine, New Haven, CT, United States

Yen Chun Tseng, PhD, University of Wisconsin–Stout, Menomonie, WI, United States

Clarissa Velázquez, BS, Illinois Institute of Technology Chicago, IL, United States

Preface

A recovery-based system of care is steeped in principles of dignity, hope, and aspiration. These are grounded in self-determination; namely, people describe for themselves their life goals and the mental health challenges and disabilities that interfere with them. People then decide among varied services, providers, and supporters (e.g., family, friends) who help them accomplish these goals. Shared decision making (SDM) is one method to do this. Briefly, *SDM* represents a helping relationship between people, their providers, and support system to help service recipients give voice to their goals and aspirations as well as barriers to them. The "shared" of SDM recognizes the existence of a significant body of information describing mental health challenges and corresponding interventions from which person-centered decision making might benefit. Providers are typically subject matter experts who educate service recipients about various options. SDM is grounded in a "counseling" relationship in which the provider then helps people weigh the pros and cons of specific decisions. Providers do this in an iterative and reflective manner oriented to assisting people to craft actions that represent their goals and aspirations.

This book represents a broad and deep dive into basic practices that compose SDM; the contributors to this volume do this by unpacking SDM in terms of its basic principles. SDM is yet another paradigmatic shift in the service system from patriarchy to recovery. When beginning my professional life over 35 years ago, I learned to view people with mental illness as victims of their illness who were often resistant to health. The doctor was the expert, and the patient was the tutee. Relationships were built on the altar of compliance, one-way guidance framed on "shoulds": Patients should take their meds or should do their rehab or should avoid alcohol. And they should be cautious not to tempt relapse by pursuing goals beyond their abilities. SDM is steeped in self-determination that frames a person's pursuit of health and life goals in terms of partnership. SDM is also down-to-earth and practical; it specifies discrete behaviors in which person and provider join together to meet personal goals.

In this book, we dissect basic SDM principles from a broader social and psychological context to better understand self-determination. For example, we consider how SDM might be used when the person is not purely rational or is coolly aloof and making decisions like an actuary. Of particular interest is broadening the focus of mental health and service decisions to reflect our diverse world. This means self-determination may have a different meaning for people who vary by ethnicity or other realities related to diversity, equity, inclusion, and accessibility—for example, by gender identity, sexual orientation, religion, age, and disability. Unfortunately, life experiences of people from marginalized groups are often affected by social disadvantages, including poverty, homelessness, and food insecurity; criminal justice involvement as a victim or an arrestee; immigration; and absence of reasonable accommodations. SDM in a broader context must include the unique intersections of individual identity.

Three areas of interest poignantly represent the experience of self-determination by diversity and marginalization. First, consider SDM for people who identify as from collective cultures, such as the Chinese culture. Western views of self-determination make the individual the sole focus of decisions. Sure, they may include personally important people, such as life partners, parents, or other family members, in the process. But when defined as partnership between person and provider, SDM falls short for more collectivist groups from East Asia, among others. Chinese individuals seeking to understand their mental health challenges, the effects of these challenges on their goals, and ways to obtain these goals despite symptoms and disabilities may feel incomplete when significant family members are absent. This is often defined by family generation when, for example, young Chinese adults with serious mental illness want to include parents in SDM. Family-centered decision making is an innovative complement to SDM discussed in this book.

Second, age at both ends of the continuum is key to experiencing SDM and self-determination. Children and young people are often trying to make sense of mental health challenges as they encounter them for the first time. In the process, they are in the midst of social and cognitive developmental tasks and experiences that provide tools to actually manage life challenges. Separation and individuation are prominent among adolescents and emerging adults. SDM requires people with serious mental illness to grapple with independence as they choose different paths to launch from the family. Parental responsibility is defined by state and federal law and by the responsibilities demanded of parents/guardians for those under 18 in the United States. The process becomes murkier as the person emerges into adulthood. Among other things, person and provider need to navigate difficult issues of empowerment: Specifically, how do providers make space for emerging adults to make decisions that seem to strain expectations? This is a system-wide task: How do mental health programs include and empower adolescents and emerging adults in SDM policies and practices?

Age is a different force at the other end of the continuum: older people with serious mental illness. Older adults have their own developmental tasks to address related to generativity and integrity. Needs related to physical illness are often added to the picture. Resources dwindle. Older people must be fully empowered for self-determination in SDM.

Third, as mentioned earlier, marginalization and social disadvantage both affect and limit SDM. Poverty significantly influences the ways in which mental health challenges are framed. The needs and goals of people with mental illness are affected by home and food insecurity. Moreover, lack of resources defined by poverty limit the range of possibilities for SDM.

WHO IS THIS BOOK FOR?

This book is written for several audiences. The depth of theory and research in this volume is intended for scholars as they approach and advance SDM. This audience may include their students who are seeking foundations in recovery-based principles and SDM. Practitioners who do SDM are equally targeted. Guidelines at the end of the book are written for them and include tools that might be pulled out and used in SDM partnerships.

OUTLINE AND ORGANIZATION

The book weaves general concepts of self-determination with the exigencies of actually doing SDM. It begins in Chapter 1 by charting where SDM falls in the evolution of a recovery-oriented care system from resistance and compliance to self-determination. SDM reflects the basics of self-determination theory (SDT). Chapter 2 comprehensively summarizes the psychological theories that underpin SDT and SDM. Chapter 3 looks more thoroughly at social determinants and disadvantages that intersect with and may undermine SDM. Chapter 4 then does a deeper dive into an especially important determinant: age. It reviews developmental theory as a way to make sense of how SDM best serves youths and young adults. SDM is rooted in recovery, and recovery has become the purview of peers and peer providers. Chapter 5 describes SDM in the emerging field of peer supporters.

Chapter 6 is written for providers, supporters, and people with lived experience as a resource to doing SDM for people with serious mental illness. It provides a step-by-step description of SDM illustrated with tables and figures as well as illustrative case example(s). It refers to worksheets available for download (from the Resources tab at https://www.apa.org/pubs/books/shared-decision-making-serious-mental-illness) for use by providers with their SDM partner—the person with lived experience. Chapter 7 ends the book by discussing how scholars and health providers can develop SDM interventions in mental health care—in collaboration with people with lived experience—and the role of community-based participatory research in this process.

Acknowledgments

My thoughts about and experiences with shared decision making (SDM) that are embedded in a recovery-oriented system have been brewing most of my professional life. I trace all of this back to 1990, when I was a postdoc for Bob Liberman at the University of California, Los Angeles and we wrote "From Noncompliance to Collaboration in the Treatment of Schizophrenia" in *Hospital and Community Psychiatry* (Corrigan et al., 1990). Bob helped me understand how dated ideas of resistance and compliance undermine a person's recovery journey. At about that time, Bill Anthony at Boston University on the other side of the continent introduced me to the emerging vision of recovery in an article (Anthony, 1993) in the *Psychosocial Rehabilitation Journal*. That article tore down Emil Kraepelin's stubborn notion of unavoidable downhill course and, instead, hosted hope and aspiration as primary.

With feedback from colleagues (Larry Davidson, Mark Salzer, Beth Angell, and Steve Marcus) at the Center on Adherence and Self-Determination, I pushed beyond noncompliance and collaboration in a 2012 article "From Adherence to Self-Determination" in *Psychiatric Services* (Corrigan et al., 2012). And between this article and Anthony's came the 2006 clarion article on SDM from Bob Drake and Pat Deegan published in *Psychiatric Services* (Deegan & Drake, 2006). My head continues to spin with the varied effects of these manuscripts on me.

My journey has been augmented closer to home with the intellectual partnership of colleagues, including Stan McCracken, Paul Holmes, Jon Larson, Nicolas Rusch, Kristin Kosyluk, and Lindsay Sheehan. I have also benefited from the wisdom of people with lived experience, including Andrea Schmuck, Bob Lundin, Sonya Ballentine, and Karyn Bolden Stovall.

REFERENCES

Anthony, W. A. (1993). Recovery from mental illness: The guiding vision of the mental health service system in the 1990s. *Psychosocial Rehabilitation Journal*, *16*(4), 11–23. https://doi.org/10.1037/h0095655

Corrigan, P. W., Angell, B., Davidson, L., Marcus, S. C., Salzer, M. S., Kottsieper, P., Larson, J. E., Mahoney, C. A., O'Connell, M. J., & Stanhope, V. (2012). From adherence to self-determination: Evolution of a treatment paradigm for people with serious mental illness. *Psychiatric Services*, *63*(2), 169–173. https://doi.org/10.1176/appi.ps.201100065

Corrigan, P. W., Liberman, R. P., & Engel, J. D. (1990). From noncompliance to collaboration in the treatment of schizophrenia. *Hospital and Community Psychiatry*, *41*(11), 1203–1211. https://doi.org/10.1176/ps.41.11.1203

Deegan, P. E., & Drake, R. E. (2006). Shared decision making and medication management in the recovery process. *Psychiatric Services*, *57*(11), 1636–1639. https://doi.org/10.1176/ps.2006.57.11.1636

SHARED DECISION MAKING AND SERIOUS MENTAL ILLNESS

1

FROM ADHERENCE TO SELF-DETERMINATION

Choosing to Participate in "My" Service Plan

PATRICK W. CORRIGAN AND VIRGINIA SPICKNALL

An evolving foundation to treatment has paralleled development and implementation of shared decision making (SDM) in the service delivery system for people with serious mental illness (SMI). It represents a journey from somewhat dated notions of patient adherence (obeying treatment prescriptions) to contemporary principles of personal determination of goals and ways to accomplish these goals. This chapter recounts the evolution from adherence to self-determination that forms the basis of SDM. We begin by briefly addressing what is meant by SMI and the evidence-based practices that help people meet their goals. We then review the body of research that shows people with SMI often choose not to participate in evidence-based practices. We detour here for a necessary discussion of how to measure lack of participation in evidence-based practices. This leads to our summary of the evolving nature of why people do not participate—for example, resistance and noncompliance. Self-determination has emerged in its place; hence, we review basic psychological theory that explains the benefits and processes of self-determination. Several strategies have gained traction for promoting self-determination in mental health service. We review these strategies and highlight the prominent role SDM has in this regard.

https://doi.org/10.1037/0000478-001
Shared Decision Making and Serious Mental Illness, P. W. Corrigan (Editor)

We define *engagement* as the ultimate purpose of strategies that promotes self-determination vis-à-vis treatment services. Engagement rests on two perspectives. First, engagement reflects a view of the person: It represents the sum of considerations and actions individuals experience in actually using evidence-based practices to meet life goals. Engagement rejects the negative valence that is sometimes suggested by not adhering: that by choosing not to do some treatment—for example, not taking one's medication, not working with the job coach, or not participating in family therapy—the person is somehow doing something wrong. This absence of adherence does not represent some kind of moral or personality flaw. Principles of engagement replace any kind of judgment about personal treatment decisions with acceptance; the provider supports personal choice.

Engagement also provides perspective about the provider team and setting, namely, whether the setting offers services that support individual goals. Hence, people may choose not to engage in a specific evidence-based approach because of the way in which it is provided. Concerns about cultural competence and humility are one factor for this disconnect. This is not necessarily meant as an indictment of specific providers or settings as much as a realization that differences between goals and settings may diminish an individual's choice to engage.

Consider the case of Janet.[1] Janet is a 33-year-old woman with schizoaffective disorder who lives in a downtown condo with her partner and is a paralegal at a large law firm. She has been taking the same antipsychotic medication and seeking services from the same provider for the past 5 years. Her symptoms include occasional distressing delusions (e.g., "Everyone knows what I am thinking") and hallucinations (e.g., hearing threatening voices). They seem to be handled well by her mix of medication, counseling, and support. Despite this, Janet is bothered at times by some of the antipsychotic medication's side effects. She occasionally experiences nausea and drowsiness that have led to her staying home from work. Her side effects are interfering with job performance. She wants to consider a change but recalls unintended results of past medicine changes that have led her physician to be conservative about such actions. What should she do?

---

[1]Case examples in this book are hypothetical.

WHAT ARE SERIOUS MENTAL ILLNESSES?

The text revision of the fifth edition of the *Diagnostic and Statistical Manual of Mental Disorders* (American Psychiatric Association, 2022) defines many syndromes as serious, including those in the schizophrenia spectrum, anxiety and affective disorders, eating disorders, posttraumatic stress disorder, and personality disorders. Janet's diagnosis of schizoaffective disorder clearly falls in this group. Clinical research has suggested, however, that it is not diagnosis per se that defines seriousness but, rather, the prolonged distress, dysfunctions, and disabilities engendered by experience with the disorder (Linden, 2017; Zimmerman et al., 2018). For example, people with seemingly less severe social anxiety disorders may experience a worse course than those with the prototypic serious illness—schizophrenia—because the fright and nervousness defining their anxiety prevents them from seeking even the least demanding of jobs, thereby rendering them unable to live on their own. Many people diagnosed with schizoaffective disorder, like Janet Williamson, can live with recurring auditory hallucinations without distress; they pursue careers and enjoy full family lives.

Dysfunctions that arise from SMI affect the four fundamental spheres of human psychology: (a) affect, (b) perception and cognition, (c) motivation and behavior, and (d) interpersonal functioning (Corrigan et al., 2008, 2024). Affect includes distress, depression, and euphoria. *Distress* is marked by rumination and autonomic reactions, whereas *depression* manifests as intense sadness, anhedonia, and vegetative signs; these are considered the uncomfortable emotions. *Euphoria* is the obverse of these two: an overwhelming sense of intense pleasure and well-being that can lead to significant risks when in the manic phase. Problems in perception and cognition are significant among psychotic disorders and include hallucinations, delusions, and formal thought disorders. People with anxiety disorders and depression may also be harmed by obsessive thoughts that lead to worry or guilt. Many people with SMI have problems with motivation and behavior. These problems may be observed as extremes: lethargic and amotivated when depressed compared with expansive engagement in risky behavior when manic. People with mania and some psychoses might also demonstrate disinhibited behaviors, including sexual or eating behaviors that are extreme for them. Interpersonal functioning is also affected for many people with SMIs. Some may not have mastered basic communication, assertiveness, or problem-solving skills necessary to meet social goals (Cotter et al., 2018; Girard et al., 2017; Speed et al., 2018).

Within these challenges to the basic psychological functions are suicide and violence, which are among the most serious consequences of mental illnesses. The 2016–2020 National Hospital Ambulatory Medical Care Survey estimated the lifetime prevalence of suicidal ideation in the United States to be 15.6% (Alexander et al., 2023). Based on the 2022 National Survey of Drug Use and Mental Health, 0.6% of the adults aged 18 or older made at least one suicide attempt, whereas the most recent Youth Risk Behaviors Survey from 2021 found that 10.0% of youths in Grades 9 through 12 reported that they had made at least one suicide attempt in the past 12 months (Substance Abuse and Mental Health Services Administration [SAMHSA], 2023b). These ratios are significantly higher when the person has an SMI: of those who died by suicide captured in the 2022 report, 90% had a diagnosable mental health condition. Globally, an estimated 703,000 people die by suicide each year (World Health Organization [WHO], 2021). Violence among people with SMI can also be concerning: Epidemiological research has suggested it might be as high as 3.6 times that of the comparable population (Thornicroft, 2020; Van Dorn et al., 2012). Suicide and violence are unlike other symptoms and dysfunctions because of their potential to cause irrevocable harm to self or others.

Distress and dysfunctions lead to disabilities, manifestations of the illness that prevent the person from achieving goals typical of their age and culture (Cree et al., 2020; Linden, 2017; Wade & Halligan, 2017). Three goals are especially relevant to a good quality of life in the Western worldview:

1. Independent living: Most adults want to start a household that represents their lifestyle. This includes decisions about place of residence, housing type, roommates/intimacy/commitment, decor, visitors, and neighborhood. It also includes basics related to food, clothing, and other manifestations of style.

2. Education and employment: Goals of independent living are more likely to be accomplished when the person has a satisfying job. Meeting higher educational standards is often needed for this kind of job. Employment also includes notions of vocation and affiliation. People want to work at places that meet their sense of achievement and that provide a satisfying interpersonal network.

3. Health: People seek good mental and physical health. Beyond health, they wish to pursue wellness, a physical and psychological robustness related to well-being and life satisfaction. Health and wellness are often affected by one's spiritual life.

WHAT ARE EVIDENCE-BASED SERVICES?

Clinical sciences and professional groups have developed and tested evidence-based practice guidelines to help people with serious psychiatric disorders manage distress and disabilities to accomplish life goals (American Psychiatric Association, n.d., 2015, 2020, 2023; American Psychological Association, n.d., 2017, 2021, 2022). Table 1.1 summarizes a number of evidence-based practices currently recognized by SAMHSA (2023a).

In 1997, SAMHSA launched the National Registry of Evidence-based Programs and Practices (NREPP) to track evidence-based services for people with SMI. The original site housed a ranking of expert-endorsed mental health and substance use-related programs and practices. NREPP was replaced

TABLE 1.1. SAMHSA-Recognized Evidence-Based Practices for the Treatment of Mental Illness and Substance Use Disorders

Evidence-based practice	Definition	Systematic review
Supported employment	An approach wherein the goal is to identify competitive employment in the community and to ensure an environment that provides for people's needs through follow-along supports	• Bond et al. (2023) • Richter & Hoffmann (2019)
ACT	A multidisciplinary, team-based service delivery model that provides time-unlimited, community-based services for individuals with SMI who experience or are at particular risk for concurrent substance use, frequent hospitalization, homelessness, involvement with the criminal legal system, and psychiatric crises; the primary goal of ACT is to help individuals achieve recovery through community treatment, rehabilitation, and support	• Arahanthabailu et al. (2023) • Cuddeback et al. (2020) • Mantzouranis et al. (2019)
Psychotropic medication	Medication that affects how the brain works and causes changes in mood, awareness, thoughts, feelings, or behavior	• Cuijpers et al. (2020) • Huang et al. (2022) • Isohanni et al. (2021)

(continues)

TABLE 1.1. SAMHSA-Recognized Evidence-Based Practices for the Treatment of Mental Illness and Substance Use Disorders (*Continued*)

Evidence-based practice	Definition	Systematic review
Psychotherapy (e.g., CBT, DBT, REBT, acceptance and commitment therapy, motivational interviewing, group therapy, family therapy)	Counseling and therapy usually focused on developing healthy skills to cope and can help one better understand the cause of their thoughts and behaviors, so they can change unhealthy patterns	• Cuijpers (2017, 2019) • Matweychuk et al. (2019) • Pace et al. (2017)
Support groups	Peer support, encompassing a range of activities and interactions among people who share similar experiences of being diagnosed with mental health conditions, substance use disorders, or both; this mutuality—often called *peerness*—between a peer support worker and person in or seeking recovery promotes connection and inspires hope	• Brunelli et al. (2016) • Shorey & Chua (2023)
Harm reduction	Engaging directly with people who use drugs to prevent overdose and infectious disease transmission; improve physical, mental, and social well-being; and offer low-barrier options for accessing health care services, including substance use and mental health disorder treatment	• Levengood et al. (2021) • O'Leary et al. (2024)

Note. SAMHSA = Substance Abuse and Mental Health Services Administration; ACT = assertive community treatment; SMI = serious mental illness; CBT = cognitive behavior therapy; DBT = dialectical behavior therapy; REBT = rational emotive behavior therapy.

by the Evidence-Based Practices Resource Center (EBPRC) in 2018 (Green-Hennessy, 2018). The aim of the EBPRC is to house evidence-based treatment improvement protocols, tool kits, resource guides, and clinical practice guidelines. The site allows users to search by topic area, substance or condition, resource type, population type (e.g., youths, adult), target audience (e.g., resource for clinicians, prevention professionals, patients, policymakers), and authoring organization.

Choosing Not to Engage in Evidence-Based Services

Of the several reasons that might explain failure of people to engage, two are considered in this section. One is the side effects of medication or psychosocial interventions, and the second is the lack of availability.

Side Effects

Side effects might dissuade a person from pursuing specific practices. Side effects are especially well examined in medications; traditional antipsychotic medication has been shown to affect every organ system deleteriously with particularly troubling effects related to movement and restlessness (Ali et al., 2021) Atypical antipsychotic medications meant to diminish these sides effects have their own troubling profile, causing, among other things, significant weight gain, which can lead to diabetes and cardiovascular disease (B. B. Barton et al., 2020) Although generally with fewer side effects, antidepressants like tricyclics and selective serotonin reuptake inhibitors may affect cognitive functioning, sleep, and libido (Wang et al., 2018). Mood stabilizers for bipolar disorder can also cause a range of unintended metabolic effects (Himmerich & Hamilton, 2022).

Although side effects are most commonly examined in terms of psychopharmacology; evidence-based practices with a psychosocial focus may yield similar unintended consequences (Crawford et al., 2016; Lönnqvist, 1985). These might include focusing on goals that are not the person's priority, demanding too much time or other resources, forestalling other interests (e.g., skills training instead of supported education), or excluding important others in the intervention process (e.g., not pursuing family interventions; Corrigan et al., 2024).

The impact of side effects is broadly evidenced across most health conditions. A Centers for Disease Control and Prevention *Morbidity and Mortality Weekly Report* published in 2017 demonstrated that physicians write 3.8 billion prescriptions every year, yet only one in five new ones ever gets filled (Neiman et al., 2017). Further, only 50% of those filled are taken correctly. A meta-analysis comprising 46 studies on adherence to psychotropic medication found similar results: Forty-nine percent of major psychiatric disorder patients chose not to engage in medication (Semahegn et al., 2020). Rates of adherence for those with schizophrenia, major depressive disorders, and bipolar disorders were 56%, 50%, and 44% respectively.

We also see adherence issues outside of medication use. For example, people routinely avoid scheduling appointments for mental health–related issues despite obtaining referrals from providers (Andrade et al., 2014; Hacker et al., 2014; Walker et al., 2015). Even once appointments are established, attrition rates are relatively high. For example, a meta-analysis comprising 20,995 participants receiving cognitive behavior therapy found treatment dropout rates to be 35% on average across 115 studies (E. Fernandez et al., 2015). A similar rate of 30.4% was found in a more recent meta-analysis done by Lappan et al. (2020) when analyzing 151 studies looking at dropout rates of in-person psychosocial substance use disorder treatments. WHO's World Mental Health Survey Initiative yielded average dropout rates of 30% from high-income countries and 45% from low- and middle-income countries for outpatient mental health care programs (D. Fernández et al., 2021). This study also determined that dropout occurs most frequently within the first two visits. Although it seems initiation and retention of mental health services pose challenges, studies also have shown that it is common for those who engage in psychiatric treatment to not complete between-session work recommended by their mental health providers, such as psychoeducational, self-assessment, and modality-specific tasks (Decker et al., 2016; Kazantzis et al., 2016; Leeuwerik et al., 2019; Tang & Kreindler, 2017). Similar issues with engagement can be found when working with people on vocational, independent living, nutrition, and exercise goals (Fahey et al., 2018; Ipsen & Goe, 2016; Lemstra et al., 2016; Mandal & Ose, 2020).

Availability

A separate category of factors that undermine engagement, which is indicative of the provider system, is that services are not available. Many urban settings, for example, lack sufficient resources to provide services throughout their metropolitan area, especially during a significant economic recession (Antunes et al., 2017; Okkels et al., 2018; Ruiz-Pérez et al., 2017). Rural settings have a separate set of hurdles that undermine availability and dissemination of services (Okkels et al., 2018). Compounding these barriers is an absence of services that represent the exigencies of cultural groups like African Americans, Asian Americans, Latinos, and Native Americans (Kirmayer & Minas, 2008; Norcross & Wampold, 2019)—for example, family involvement in treatment decisions.

Some services are available but are not faithful to evidence-based protocol. Evidence-based psychosocial practices include clear principles and strategies necessary to accomplish the goals of such practice. Unfortunately, measures of service fidelity often show providers lack training to do the evidence-based practice or stray from the manual once implemented in a real-world setting (Fonagy & Luyten, 2019; Prowse et al., 2015). The unavailability of high-quality services influences personal attitudes about services, often causing people to become more pessimistic about possible benefits. Although unavailable services are a compelling concern, it is still clear that choosing not to participate is an individual and powerful cause of nonadherence.

Defining the Problem More Objectively

Attendance is one seemingly easy-to-assess way in which service participation has been construed—for example, does the person show up at weekly scheduled sessions? Although face-to-face meetings may be important, what the person does in the interim is probably more essential to progress. This might be called *homework*, goal-related efforts the person has attempted outside of the treatment setting. Attendance and homework can be surprisingly complex constructs despite the seeming ease in which they are represented as quantity and pattern over time. Quantity, for example, may be simply assessed as hours a week for individual psychotherapy. Most evidence-based practices, however, are not based on such narrow constrictions. For example, participation in evidence-based practices like assertive community treatment (ACT) needs broader indices because the service may be provided in short 20-minute spurts for months or even years. Moreover, many long-term evidence-based practices are not described by linear, continuous patterns. Service consumers may come and go from ACT as their current goals dictate.

Service decisions and behaviors are often centered in interactions that are described as qualities of the person–provider relationship that facilitate experience with the evidence-based practice. Much of this research has focused on qualities of the service provider, but the interest here is a bit different, centering on characteristics of the interaction. Do people, for example, find the exchange satisfying and relevant to their needs (Barkham et al., 2021)? *Trust*—defined as an emotional connection in which the person feels hopeful that the service provider is directing efforts to jointly address the issues of concern (Krupnik, 2023)—is one important way in which satisfying relationships have been studied. Service interactions are often construed as simple, one-to-one exchanges. In reality, many evidence-based practices are provided by teams of providers comprising individuals who vary in discipline and status (e.g., the psychiatrist focusing on medication vs. the paraprofessional providing daily ACT).

The diversity of service agents needs to be considered when assessing consumer interaction relevant to self-determination and service decisions. Peer-provided evidence-based practices have emerged as an especially important way to enhance interactions (Corrigan, 2021; Shin & Choi, 2020; White et al., 2020). Of their many benefits, peer-provided services highlight another important characteristic of interactions: their level of formality or lack thereof. More classic psychotherapies have trained practitioners for formal, sometimes aloof relationships. Providers of ACT and supported employment tend to demonstrate more informal and immediate interactions. Peer-provider exchanges are less often dictated by preconceived theory but, instead, are directed by the seemingly spontaneous demands of the moment.

Still, research begs the question: What is the metric that shows whether specific decisions and behaviors are helpful, beneficial, or otherwise positive? This is an important question for methodological as well as theoretical reasons. Researchers need to move the dependent variable in research on health decisions and behaviors from categorical indices (yes or no; did the patient decide to take the medication?) to a more statistically powerful and continuous one. Because the focus here is on self-determined medication, a Likert scale of relevance might be various conceptualizations of satisfaction with health decisions and behaviors. Satisfaction might be more fully understood in terms of a hierarchy for evaluating treatments: symptom remission, disability adjustment, goal attainment, and quality of life (Liberman, 2008; Miglietta et al., 2018). Psychiatry had traditionally restricted assessment of medication to symptom remission: Did the person administering antidepressant medication show remitted sadness and anhedonia? With many chronic symptoms comes disability—for example, the person who is unable to work because of severe and chronic depression. Hence, did treatment lead to less dysfunction and better ability to work, live independently, and enjoy intimate relationships? Functioning gains further meaning when framed in terms of personal goals—for example, did the person return to work? At the end of the day, all these constructs are important in terms of quality of life: Do people have a sense of well-being as a result of their health decisions and behaviors? Only the person seeking care can determine the importance of these spheres in assessing their health decisions.

We do not mean to be cavalier—to seemingly dismiss the benefits of traditional medicine and its body of research or ignore harmful outcomes of some medication decisions. Sometimes replacing adherence with treatment satisfaction seems to minimize the complexity of the phenomenon. As such, decisional satisfaction and behavioral satisfaction, and their juxtaposition to treatment decisions, describe a complex area of theory and method development, a topic we have tackled elsewhere (Corrigan et al., 2024). There are, for example, disease processes that confound the decisions and behavior, such as the thought disorders of some psychiatric illnesses; see Chapter 2, this volume. In absence of conditions like these, however, it seems like only the person can judge the trade-off of increased symptoms, unintended consequences, and overall well-being. Satisfaction is the juxtaposition of the costs and benefits of health decisions, the heart of the rational patient model discussed later in this book.

WHY PEOPLE CHOOSE NOT TO PARTICIPATE

Psychiatry providers have posited various reasons why people choose not to participate in treatment, leading to a winding road of essentially disempowering views about decision making (see Figure 1.1). This road is framed as a progression from relatively patriarchal and aloof notions that people failing treatment are resisting to perspectives centered around partnership and collaboration to the current evolution of self-determination that best reflects and shepherds a person's recovery. Self-development as both principle and practice fits between collaboration and self-determination. People who did not participate in services were believed to be resisting care and risking symptom remission and relapse. Some intrapsychic processes were hypothesized to block the person from fully engaging in treatment (Messer, 2002); they were mostly ego-protective factors that developed from early interactions with significant others. Many psychoanalytic theorists have expressed the belief that examination of resistance is a central core of the therapeutic process (Adler & Bachant, 1998; H. S. Gill, 1988). Although these ideas may seem out of date, there are still practitioners who view working through treatment resistance as important to care (Siegel et al., 2017; Stivers &

FIGURE 1.1. The Winding Road That Represents Personal Decision Making

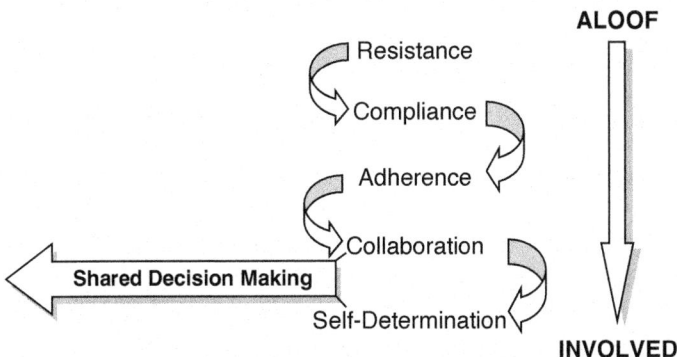

Timmermans, 2020), including services for people with psychosis (Sweeney et al., 2015). It was the risk of relapse that metaphorically set off an alarm for aggressive intervention.

Some theorists have tried to transcend seemingly accusatory notions behind resistance and have transitioned into ideas of compliance. Compliance was meant more as an objective indicator—a categorical assessment: yes or no—regarding whether the person has taken medications or otherwise participated in treatment as prescribed (Vuckovich, 2010). Treatment failure—for example, not taking one's medication—can lead to some kind of irreversible tragedy like suicide. Concerns about compliance led researchers into a useful search for unbiased and sensitive measures of whether people were participating in treatment as written by their physicians (Velligan et al., 2010). For some, compliance meant people doing their treatment regardless of its effect on self-determination. Hence, strategies meant to serve compliance have included inpatient and outpatient commitment, more benign coercion (e.g., exercise of a guardian's authority), diminished personal control (e.g., depot injections of antipsychotic medication), or benevolent trickery (e.g., not sharing the full range of side effects; Burns, 2009; Redlich et al., 2006; Szasz, 2007).

Adherence followed compliance: Practitioners defined active participation in treatment decisions, rather than actual actions, as the goal. This was partly meant to reflect an ethical perspective—that by virtue of their humanity, service recipients are due agency over their lives (Rudnick, 2008a, 2008b). Partly, this was also recognition of basic behavioral science. People will retreat from social exchanges of any kind in which a specific behavior is forced on them in a sort of "don't tell me what to think" phenomenon (Jonas et al., 2009; C. H. Miller & Quick, 2010; Quick & Stephenson, 2008). Adherence is a call to service providers for the active participation of people with mental illnesses in their care. Service providers might still dominate in developing treatment goals but seek to involve individuals with SMIs when possible.

Collaboration recognizes the expertise in the person and care provider—that, for example, the psychiatrist is expert in symptoms and biological processes whereas the person is expert in their own illness, the life in which the illness plays out, and previous treatments that have helped or have caused unintended side effects. The idea of collaboration was an insightful perspective for its time, elevating the patient to equal status with the provider and, through this peer relationship as it were, generating the most effective plan. This reflects the basics of SDM, namely that the provider partners with the person to develop and implement effective treatment plans. Self-determination enhances the person's role in this partnership. The ultimate worth of goals and interventions rests in the person's perspective. Hence, ultimately, person and provider may not be partners. Regardless of provider insight and wisdom, people decide among SDM-derived options what works best for them.

SELF-DETERMINATION IN A RECOVERY-ORIENTED CARE SYSTEM

Principles that matured in person-centered service systems add additional conceptual perspective for self-determination and decision making. These include ideas related to recovery and hope, empowerment, and personal responsibility.

Recovery and Hope

Recovery

> refers to the process in which people are able to live, work, learn, and participate fully in their communities. For some individuals, recovery is the ability to live a fulfilling and productive life despite a disability. For others, recovery implies the reduction or complete remission of symptoms. (Hogan, 2003, p. 5; see also Davidson et al., 2021, and Slade & Longden, 2015)

Classic notions of mental illness, best represented by Kraepelin's (1919) dementia praecox, described schizophrenia, for example, as marked by a progressive downhill course and suggested that treatment should be focused on realistic expectations of never being able to live independently, work, marry, or have children. Long-term follow-up studies, however, have not supported this pessimism. Many people with mental illness are able to live a high-quality life outside the mental health system (Calabrese & Corrigan, 2005; Leonhardt et al., 2017). This has led to psychiatric services that now foster hope in terms of attaining the person's goals. Recovery reintroduces ideas of the future and aspiration to describing SMI. In hope is the idea of goals and attainment, which emerged as a mental health priority largely from person-led movements with the motto "Nothing About Us Without Us" (Chamberlin, 1978).

Personal Empowerment

Out of recovery has come the call for empowerment. Some people believe personal empowerment and self-determination are different sides of the same coin (Sprague & Hayes, 2000). Research studies have unpacked the complexity of empowerment and found it to include five recurring themes: (a) self-efficacy and self-esteem, (b) powerlessness, (c) optimism/control over future, (d) righteous anger, and (e) group/community action (Rogers et al., 1997, 2010). A hierarchical factor analysis showed these constructs actually represent two higher order concepts that serve as excellent foci for self-determination: self- versus community orientations to personal empowerment (Corrigan et al., 1999). A *self-orientation* reflects the ideas of personal agency and confidence in deciding about and following through on goals and choices: What must the person have in place to successfully determine their directions? A *community orientation* redirects the lens of determination: What must the system do to make sure people have power over their choices? Self-determination is promoted by helping people grasp personal empowerment for themselves and by directing the community not to throw up barriers to the process.

Personal Responsibility

Self-determination is not meant as carte blanche for the pursuit of personal goals. Self-determination of people with SMIs needs to be understood in terms of limits experienced by most adults. No one can expect all goals to be achievable without an effect on others or that the person should be able to achieve an aspiration regardless of real-world demands. The public generally expects people will make decisions that reflect not only their interest, but those of other important people, such as friends and family, with, perhaps most prominent here, being one's spouse or children. The idea of responsibility might be viewed as a restraint to self-determination—that people are responsible for partaking in treatment so as not to burden others. We believe the idea of responsibility is empowering; indeed, many advocates for the recovery movement outline the key role of personal accountability (Price-Robertson et al., 2017; Slade, 2009). Personal accountability suggests that people with mental illness are just like others: capable of making righteous choices and therefore deserving of self-determination.

Still, at the end of the day, people with SMIs must identify for themselves their goals of the moment given external pressures. This means they consider who is important in their network and what is the relative value of specific goals as long as these considerations of one's network and goals do not supersede minimum social assumptions as laid out in criminal and civil statutes. It seems reasonable, for example, that a woman moves out on her husband when that spouse has physically abused her. Less support would be found for the father moving out on his young children because he wants to return to trade school. Self-determination requires a balanced perspective, exercising one's personal agency while responsibly considering the concerns of important others.

WAYS TO PROMOTE SELF-DETERMINATION

We limit this section to examine a proposed dichotomy of engagement highlighted earlier: (a) what can be done to help people understand options, make decisions, and act on these decisions and (b) how the community and clinic might facilitate this process while tearing down barriers to self-determined options. SDM is the best paradigm for the first, whereas community-level considerations that promote unencumbered health decisions reflect the second.

The Power of Shared Decision Making

Although the basics of SDM are described more fully throughout this book, it's important at this stage to know that SDM is a fairly well-developed and evaluated approach to health options that combines three basic principles and strategies: (a) cost–benefit analyses, (b) education, and (c) support (Drake et al., 2010). The primary goal here is to assist people in making decisions by helping them examine costs and benefits of health options and life goals. Namely, people are encouraged to identify and make sense of the advantages and disadvantages of the interventions that lead to achieving specific goals. This cost–benefit analysis is facilitated by information that aids people in better understanding life goals vis-à-vis health challenges, corresponding interventions, and other relevant parameters.

The education process requires the development of meaningful and user-friendly information channels. These might include face-to-face classroom kinds of endeavors or online technologies, such as interactive websites and social media forums (Bevan Jones et al., 2018; Naslund et al., 2016; Seyedfatemi et al., 2021). Health-related decision making is fundamentally social intercourse between person and provider. Skills that enhance the qualities of the exchange positively affect treatment decisions. This consideration has been prominently incorporated in motivational interviewing, suggesting SDM exchanges need to sidestep some kind of actuarial process to include empathy, genuineness, and the promotion of self-efficacy (Elwyn et al., 2016; W. R. Miller & Rose, 2010). Meaningful and genuine exchanges like these can provide a sense of support for individuals involved in treatment. In the process of SDM, the support offered can be both instrumental and emotional. The balance between these types of support may vary depending on the needs and goals of the person receiving treatment, the service organization, and the type of provider involved.

Research has examined SDM for a variety of illnesses and disabilities, including treatment decisions related to cancer (Herrera et al., 2023; Martínez-González et al., 2018), heart disease (Mitropoulou et al., 2023), prostatic hypertrophy (Ngu et al., 2022), mental illness (Alguera-Lara et al., 2017; Slade, 2017; Thomas et al., 2021; Zisman-Ilani et al., 2021), substance abuse (Friedrichs et al., 2016; Marchand et al., 2019), and gastrointestinal disorders (Fox & Lipstein, 2020; Song & Wu, 2022). Meta-analyses and reviews of studies have yielded mixed conclusions (Austin et al., 2015; Shay & Lafata, 2015). Findings from randomized clinical trials (RCTs) showed SDM leads to enhanced satisfaction with and more knowledge about treatments and their providers. However, findings are mixed at best about whether SDM leads to a meaningful increase of treatment-related behaviors. Perhaps one reason SDM is limited for people with SMIs is the effect of their cognitive deficits. As a result of information-processing dysfunctions, some people are unable to understand the balance of advantages and disadvantages of specific health decisions. Toward this end, cognitive therapies have been developed and tested to enhance a person's treatment decisions and behaviors. Although some of these therapies have targeted thought contents (e.g., inaccurate beliefs about the harm of a medication), in the Beckian approach to cognitive behavior therapy—that is, challenging irrational thoughts that undermine some health decisions (Aguirre Velasco et al., 2020)—what has been more successful are cognitive rehabilitation attempts to diminish the processing deficits that undermine comprehension of these decisions. Cognitive adaptation training (CAT) is a good example that has a growing set of supporting evidence (Allott et al., 2020; Velligan et al., 2015, 2023). One-way cognitive rehabilitation addresses information-processing deficits is by providing tasks that exercise key processes, such as attention and memory (Reser et al., 2019). CAT is an example of the alternative, seemingly more effective, approach to cognitive rehabilitation—namely, the provision of compensatory strategies and environmental supports specifically built around real-world tasks of the individual. To help people with cognitive difficulties that result from SMI, they might work with a service provider, for example, to clear out old prescriptions and over-the-counter medications from the bathroom cabinet; set all current prescriptions in an organized, daily pill box; and record a message in the person's own voice tied to a computer alarm that reminds them "it's time to take my medication."

Removal of Situational or Contextual Barriers to Self-Determination

Another set of approaches to enhancing SDM needs to identify and erase contextual hurdles to self-determination. Three ways of doing that are considered here: (a) educating stakeholders about the ethics and realities of self-determination, (b) reducing legislation and other government activities that restrict health decisions, and (c) streamlining interventions so participating in them is not onerous. Removing the hurdles is not enough, however. Policies and actions that encourage and support self-determination are equally important.

Education About Self-Determination

There is evidence that stakeholders are learning about recovery and ideas of self-determination it promotes. People with mental illnesses have been at the forefront of recovery, and research suggests more individuals with psychiatric disabilities are understanding and endorsing this perspective (White et al., 2020). More recently, family members have joined the movement (Corrigan & Lee, 2021; van Nistelrooij et al., 2017). Service providers seem to be last in their recognition and agreement (Hajizadeh et al., 2015). Still, there is sobering evidence of a seniority effect in some professions: Those practicing in the field longer are less likely to endorse ideas of recovery and self-determination. Many professional training programs have incorporated recovery and people in recovery into their training programs to stimulate interest in and educate newer generations of psychiatrists in the treatment paradigm shift (Gambino et al., 2016; Hornik-Lurie et al., 2018). Some evidence has suggested that endorsing recovery is associated with strengths-based approaches and community-based psychiatric rehabilitation (Thornicroft et al., 2016; Tse et al., 2016).

Laws and Policies That Promote Recovery

Education does not always lead to change in treatment behavior. Hence, efforts have been made to codify principles of recovery. In part, this has been vigorously debated in legislation related to such diverse issues as outpatient commitment (Enriquez, 2019; Thornicroft & Henderson, 2016) and psychiatric advanced directives (Belanger, 2017). More immediate to the mental health system than activities of the legislature are policies of the executive branch of government. The New Freedom Commission on Mental Health (2003) rested its 2003 report to the U.S. president based on a recovery-oriented system (Hogan, 2003). Other countries have joined the effort, too, including England, Australia, New Zealand, and the Netherlands (Craig, 2008; Davidson et al., 2008; Pilgrim, 2008). Most individual states have followed suit; specific examples of a recovery orientation have included meaningful consumer and family involvement in government decisions, especially in terms of new spending; support of consumer-developed and consumer-operated services; consumer-responsive crisis planning and advance directives; and statewide recovery education programs (R. Barton, 1998; K. J. Gill, 2006; Jacobson & Curtis, 2000).

Convenience and Immediacy

Some services unintentionally throw up barriers because they are cumbersome, thus demanding time or resources that exceed personal limits. Service providers have sought to make specific practices more convenient. Framing this as convenience might seem to minimize their importance, but humans as a whole choose behaviors with the least demands. Hence, practical, grassroots approaches to services have emerged. Some are obvious from where we sit today: Move services out of the office and beyond the 9-to-5 workday to offer assistance when and where the person needs it. No longer is the aim of treatment to obtain insight into a problem or learn social skills for difficult interactions. Instead, they are more obvious and immediate: Help the person get to the physician to investigate their chest cold or cash the social security check for today's groceries. The provider might actually get involved in these services. They might, for example, help the person make a schedule for taking the day's prescribed medications. This is an especially poignant and timely process for services meant to address people with SMIs who are homeless (Kaduszkiewicz et al., 2017; Upshur et al., 2018) or court involved (Horst et al., 2023; Munthe et al., 2016).

CULTURAL ADAPTATIONS OF SDM

SDM and self-determination with its base in competence and autonomy may stereotypically reflect individualist priorities of Western countries that may be foreign to some East Asian groups (Lee et al., 2015). Cultural values of autonomy, for example, seem contrary to those of relatedness and group cohesion (Iyengar & Lepper, 1999). Adopting choices made by trusted others uniquely enhances intrinsic motivation for many East Asian individuals. In this light, it makes sense that many East Asian patients living in the United States may more actively involve family members in decision-making efforts. Research has shown, for example, that family dynamics may supersede self-care concerns among many Asian Americans (Cho et al., 2015). Specific dynamics among some Chinese patients seem to include the essential importance of family, deference to authority figures, maintenance of interpersonal harmony, and self-restraint (Lee et al., 2015).

Family-Centered Decision Making

There is a growing body of work on family-centered decision making (FCDM) for adults with SMI. The central question here is whether and how much family members, especially parents, should be actively involved in health care decision making. One study showed that a group of Korean American patients with cancer significantly preferred active family involvement in care-seeking compared with European American patients (Blackhall et al., 1995). Another study with a Southeast Asian sample showed that proponents of FCDM might favor withholding information from family members with cancer (Back & Huak, 2005). Researchers have also identified the importance of FCDM among some East Asians related to mental health care. For example, Chinese versus American preference for decision-making types was examined in a vignette study that described two approaches for Lily, a 30-year old woman with symptoms of depression (Gao et al., 2019): (a) SDM in which Lily is fully informed about interventions, weighs the costs and benefits of her options, and makes decisions and (b) FCDM in which Lily and her parents are informed about interventions, consider the pros and cons, and then her parents make the decisions. Results showed that European Americans viewed SDM as significantly more preferable than FCDM for Lily, whereas Chinese and Chinese Americans preferred FCDM.

Developing a manualized approach is an important next step, assuming research continues to support FCDM for significant groups of East Asian patients and their families. Such manuals have already been developed and tested for SDM (Agency for Healthcare Research and Quality, 2014) and may provide a preliminary framework for the development of FCDM. The SDM manual includes educating patients about illness and treatment options, helping them consider pros and cons of individual options, and teaching the provider basic counseling skills that facilitate this interaction. Although many of these principles and practices would seem equally important for FCDM, challenges may emerge in adapting the SDM manual to family-centered practices. The decision-making process needs to be better unpacked, especially when multiple family members are concerned. How, for example, might a list of pros and cons be generated, and who might direct the process? Is consensus a useful paradigm for translating costs and benefits into a decision? How are values of age and authority as well as corresponding deference understood in the process? What if there are attitudinal issues among family toward the service provider? What is the role of the service provider in these dynamics?

Further Considerations

Despite FCDM's intuitive appeal, we need to revisit heterogeneity to further understand its effect. We do not mean to imply that all East Asian psychiatric patients, for example, would opt for FCDM in their mental health care. For example, the Gao et al. (2019) study showed acculturated Chinese—those living in America at the time of the study—were more likely to endorse SDM. Moreover, groups from other cultures may prefer FCDM. For example, research among Latinx individuals has described *familismo* (familism) and *respeto* (respect; Escobedo et al., 2018) as values that are likely to influence family roles in health decision making. Deference shown by adult children to their parents may affect choices about the child's health services. For that matter, service providers should not assume that European Americans, by virtue of their culture, will prefer SDM. Family-centeredness is likely to vary among patients of Western European heritage.

FCDM processes might vary by other social determinants, including gender and age of family member. For example, in many East Asian families, men are more typically viewed as family authorities than women (Qin & Chang, 2012). Hence, fathers may be viewed as more influential in health decisions, whereas actions based on those decisions may be carried out by mothers. Also, health decisions will change as adult children assume responsibility for health care of older parents with disabilities. Children, for example, might decide not to share diagnoses with parents challenged by a serious illness with poor prognosis. Male children may be most influential in these kinds of decisions. Interest in FCDM may vary by psychiatric diagnosis. Perhaps FCDM will be of greater priority for patients challenged by more disabling illnesses, such as schizophrenia.

Further, FCDM is not a monolithic experience. Although the development of an FCDM manual will inform providers how to engage patients in this form of decision making, it does not necessarily prescribe a portfolio of required steps. For example, patient and family may wish to limit the breadth of decisions or change family roles as illness moves from acute to relatively remitted phases, an experience that frames FCDM as a dynamic process; namely, individual patients change preferences over the course of illness and treatment. In the process, providers should remember that SDM and FCDM are not independent and static processes. Treatment may involve a continually changing mix of both two perspectives.

Patients, families, and providers should also be alert to potential negative consequences of FCDM. For example, bias, stigma, or language barriers may lead some family members to call for deferring treatment participation even when not in the patient's best interest. The choice between SDM and FCDM may also require ethical consideration. What happens, for example, if a patient and their family members disagree about the family's participation in decision making? As psychiatry has evolved, cognizance of the cultural lens in the interpretation of ethical provider behavior has increased (Okasha et al., 2008). Still, our interpretation of the Principles of Medical Ethics with annotations for psychiatry (American Psychiatric Association, 2013) prioritizes patient choice except when patients are under age of adulthood or currently dangerous to self or others. Mental health providers ultimately need to promote patient choice but seek to do so with some attention to cultural influence.

What Does the Research Say?

Although FCDM makes intuitive sense, we are surprised by the relative dearth of papers in the professional literature specific to that topic. Indeed, the handful of studies summarized here were among the few we found in the literature. This state of affairs begs for more studies, and investigations might consider two priorities. First, research should further explain preferences for SDM and FCDM and how heterogeneity of culture affects those preferences. The dynamic and mediating effects of social determinants and psychiatric diagnosis need to be included in this work. Second, effects of FCDM per se should be examined. This requires an FCDM manual and fidelity measure that could be the focus of RCTs. These RCTs may also look at feasibility, fidelity, and acceptability as well as effects on health and recovery. Assuming first-generation studies of FCDM are successful, subsequent research should identify individual differences that would help providers tailor FCDM for the patient's experience.

CONCLUSION

Personal control of one's service plan has evolved from problematic ideas that characterize people as unable to think clearly and act accordingly to those that rest on self-determination and the recovery it implies. Cultural views of self-determination need to be considered here, especially in terms of roles families might play in SDM. The goal throughout the remainder of this book is to foster a better understanding of actions that promote self-determination throughout recovery-based systems. This becomes a priority in ongoing research meant to enhance care-seeking as well as training programs for providers at the base of this system.

REFERENCES

Adler, E., & Bachant, J. L. (1998). *Working in depth: A clinician's guide to framework and flexibility in the analytic relationship.* Jason Aronson.

Agency for Healthcare Research and Quality. (2014). *The SHARE Approach: Essential steps of shared decision making.* https://www.ahrq.gov/health-literacy/professional-training/shared-decision/tools/share-poster.html

Aguirre Velasco, A., Cruz, I. S. S., Billings, J., Jimenez, M., & Rowe, S. (2020). What are the barriers, facilitators and interventions targeting help-seeking behaviours for common mental health problems in adolescents? A systematic review. *BMC Psychiatry, 20*(1), Article 293. https://doi.org/10.1186/s12888-020-02659-0

Alexander, S., Christopher, C., & Ashman, J. J. (2023). *Emergency department visits with suicidal ideation: United States, 2016–2020* (NCHS Data Brief No. 463). Centers for Disease Control and Prevention. https://doi.org/10.15620/cdc:125704

Alguera-Lara, V., Dowsey, M. M., Ride, J., Kinder, S., & Castle, D. (2017). Shared decision making in mental health: The importance for current clinical practice. *Australasian Psychiatry, 25*(6), 578–582. https://doi.org/10.1177/1039856217734711

Ali, T., Sisay, M., Tariku, M., Mekuria, A. N., & Desalew, A. (2021). Antipsychotic-induced extrapyramidal side effects: A systematic review and meta-analysis of observational studies. *PLOS ONE, 16*(9), Article e0257129. https://doi.org/10.1371/journal.pone.0257129

Allott, K., van-der-El, K., Bryce, S., Parrish, E. M., McGurk, S. R., Hetrick, S., Bowie, C. R., Kidd, S., Hamilton, M., Killackey, E., & Velligan, D. (2020). Compensatory interventions for cognitive impairments in psychosis: A systematic review and meta-analysis. *Schizophrenia Bulletin, 46*(4), 869–883. https://doi.org/10.1093/schbul/sbz134

American Psychiatric Association. (n.d.). *Clinical practice guidelines.* https://www.psychiatry.org/psychiatrists/practice/clinical-practice-guidelines#:~:text=APA%20Clinical%20Practice%20Guidelines%20provide,strategies%20in%20a%20standardized%20format

American Psychiatric Association. (2013). *The principles of medical ethics: With annotations especially applicable to psychiatry.* https://www.psychiatry.org/getmedia/3fe5eae9-3df9-4561-a070-84a009c6c4a6/2013-APA-Principles-of-Medical-Ethics.pdf

American Psychiatric Association. (2015). *Practice guidelines for the psychiatric evaluation of adults* (3rd ed.). https://doi.org/10.1176/appi.books.9780890426760

American Psychiatric Association. (2020). *The American Psychiatric Association practice guideline for the treatment of patients with schizophrenia* (3rd ed.). https://doi.org/10.1176/appi.books.9780890424841

American Psychiatric Association. (2022). *Diagnostic and statistical manual of mental disorders* (5th ed., text rev.). https://doi.org/10.1176/appi.books.9780890425787

American Psychiatric Association. (2023). *The American Psychiatric Association practice guideline for the treatment of patients with eating disorders* (4th ed.). https://doi.org/10.1176/appi.books.9780890424865

American Psychological Association. (n.d.). *APA professional practice guidelines.* https://www.apa.org/practice/guidelines

American Psychological Association. (2017). *Professional practice guidelines for integrating the role of work and career into psychological practice.* https://www.apa.org/practice/guidelines/role-work-career

American Psychological Association. (2021). *APA guidelines on evidence-based psychological practice in health care.* https://www.apa.org/about/policy/psychological-practice-health-care.pdf

American Psychological Association. (2022). *Guidelines for psychological practice in health care delivery systems.* https://www.apa.org/practice/guidelines/delivery-systems

Andrade, L. H., Alonso, J., Mneimneh, Z., Wells, J. E., Al-Hamzawi, A., Borges, G., Bromet, E., Bruffaerts, R., de Girolamo, G., de Graaf, R., Florescu, S., Gureje, O., Hinkov, H. R., Hu, C., Huang, Y., Hwang, I., Jin, R., Karam, E. G., Kovess-Masfety, V., . . . Kessler, R. C. (2014). Barriers to mental health treatment: Results from the WHO World Mental Health surveys. *Psychological Medicine, 44*(6), 1303–1317. https://doi.org/10.1017/S0033291713001943

Antunes, A., Frasquilho, D., Cardoso, G., Pereira, N., Silva, M., Caldas-de-Almeida, J. M., & Ferrão, J. (2017). Perceived effects of the economic recession on population mental health, well-being and provision of care by primary care users and professionals: A qualitative study protocol in Portugal. *BMJ Open, 7*(9), Article e017032. https://doi.org/10.1136/bmjopen-2017-017032

Arahanthabailu, P., Praharaj, S. K., Purohith, A. N., Yesodharan, R., Bhandary, R. P., & Sharma, P. S. V. N. (2023). Madison to Manipal: A narrative review of modified assertive community treatment programs. *Asian Journal of Psychiatry, 88*, Article 103746. https://doi.org/10.1016/j.ajp.2023.103746

Austin, C. A., Mohottige, D., Sudore, R. L., Smith, A. K., & Hanson, L. C. (2015). Tools to promote shared decision making in serious illness: A systematic review. *JAMA Internal Medicine, 175*(7), 1213–1221. https://doi.org/10.1001/jamainternmed.2015.1679

Back, M. F., & Huak, C. Y. (2005). Family centred decision making and non-disclosure of diagnosis in a South East Asian oncology practice. *Psycho-Oncology, 14*(12), 1052–1059. https://doi.org/10.1002/pon.918

Barkham, M., Lutz, W., & Castonguay, L. G. (2021). *Bergin and Garfield's handbook of psychotherapy and behavior change.* John Wiley & Sons.

Barton, B. B., Segger, F., Fischer, K., Obermeier, M., & Musil, R. (2020). Update on weight-gain caused by antipsychotics: A systematic review and meta-analysis. *Expert Opinion on Drug Safety, 19*(3), 295–314. https://doi.org/10.1080/14740338.2020.1713091

Barton, R. (1998). The rehabilitation-recovery paradigm: A statement of philosophy for a public mental health system. *Psychiatric Rehabilitation Skills, 2*(2), 171–187. https://doi.org/10.1080/10973435.1998.10387561

Belanger, E. (2017). Shared decision-making in palliative care: Research priorities to align care with patients' values. *Palliative Medicine, 31*(7), 585–586. https://doi.org/10.1177/0269216317713864

Bevan Jones, R., Thapar, A., Rice, F., Beeching, H., Cichosz, R., Mars, B., Smith, D. J., Merry, S., Stallard, P., Jones, I., Thapar, A. K., & Simpson, S. A. (2018). A web-based psychoeducational intervention for adolescent depression: Design and development of MoodHwb. *JMIR Mental Health, 5*(1), Article e13. https://doi.org/10.2196/mental.8894

Blackhall, L. J., Murphy, S. T., Frank, G., Michel, V., & Azen, S. (1995). Ethnicity and attitudes toward patient autonomy. *JAMA, 274*(10), 820–825. https://doi.org/10.1001/jama.1995.03530100060035

Bond, G. R., Al-Abdulmunem, M., Marbacher, J., Christensen, T. N., Sveinsdottir, V., & Drake, R. E. (2023). A systematic review and meta-analysis of IPS supported employment for young adults with mental health conditions. *Administration and Policy in Mental Health, 50*(1), 160–172. https://doi.org/10.1007/s10488-022-01228-9

Brunelli, A. A., Murphy, G. C., & Athanasou, J. A. (2016). Effectiveness of social support group interventions for psychosocial outcomes: A meta-analytic review. *Australian Journal of Rehabilitation Counselling, 22*(2), 104–127. https://doi.org/10.1017/jrc.2016.9

Burns, T. (2009). Knowledge about antipsychotic long-acting injections: Bridging that gap. *The British Journal of Psychiatry, 195*(Suppl. 52), S5–S6. https://doi.org/10.1192/bjp.195.52.s5

Calabrese, J. D., & Corrigan, P. W. (2005). Beyond dementia praecox: Findings from long-term follow-up studies of schizophrenia. In R. O. Ralph & P. W. Corrigan (Eds.), *Recovery in mental illness: Broadening our understanding of wellness* (pp. 63–84). American Psychological Association. https://doi.org/10.1037/10848-003

Chamberlin, J. (1978). *On our own: Patient-controlled alternatives to the mental health system*. McGraw-Hill.

Cho, N. H., Kim, K. M., Choi, S. H., Park, K. S., Jang, H. C., Kim, S. S., Sattar, N., & Lim, S. (2015). High blood pressure and its association with incident diabetes over 10 years in the Korean Genome and Epidemiology Study (KoGES). *Diabetes Care, 38*(7), 1333–1338. https://doi.org/10.2337/dc14-1931

Corrigan, P. W. (2021). *The power of peer providers in mental health services*. Nova Science Publishers. https://novapublishers.com/shop/the-power-of-peer-providers-in-mental-health-services/

Corrigan, P. W., Faber, D., Rashid, F., & Leary, M. (1999). The construct validity of empowerment among consumers of mental health services. *Schizophrenia Research, 38*(1), 77–84. https://doi.org/10.1016/S0920-9964(98)00180-7

Corrigan, P. W., & Lee, E.-J. (2021). Family-centered decision making for East Asian adults with mental illness. *Psychiatric Services, 72*(1), 114–116. https://doi.org/10.1176/appi.ps.201900570

Corrigan, P. W., Mueser, K. T., Bond, G. R., Drake, R. E., & Solomon, P. (2008). *Principles and practice of psychiatric rehabilitation: An empirical approach*. The Guilford Press.

Corrigan, P. W., Rüsch, N., Watson, A. C., Kosyluk, K., & Sheehan, L. (2024). *Principles and practice of psychiatric rehabilitation: Promoting recovery and self-determination* (3rd ed.). The Guilford Press.

Cotter, J., Granger, K., Backx, R., Hobbs, M., Looi, C. Y., & Barnett, J. H. (2018). Social cognitive dysfunction as a clinical marker: A systematic review of meta-analyses across 30 clinical conditions. *Neuroscience & Biobehavioral Reviews, 84*, 92–99. https://doi.org/10.1016/j.neubiorev.2017.11.014

Craig, T. J. (2008). Recovery: Say what you mean and mean what you say. *Journal of Mental Health, 17*(2), 125–128. https://doi.org/10.1080/09638230802003800

Crawford, M. J., Thana, L., Farquharson, L., Palmer, L., Hancock, E., Bassett, P., Clarke, J., & Parry, G. D. (2016). Patient experience of negative effects of psychological treatment: Results of a national survey. *The British Journal of Psychiatry*, *208*(3), 260–265. https://doi.org/10.1192/bjp.bp.114.162628

Cree, R. A., Okoro, C. A., Zack, M. M., & Carbone, E. (2020). Frequent mental distress among adults, by disability status, disability type, and selected characteristics—United States, 2018. *Morbidity and Mortality Weekly Report*, *69*(36), 1238–1243. https://doi.org/10.15585/mmwr.mm6936a2

Cuddeback, G. S., Simpson, J. M., & Wu, J. C. (2020). A comprehensive literature review of forensic assertive community treatment (FACT): Directions for practice, policy and research. *International Journal of Mental Health*, *49*(2), 106–127. https://doi.org/10.1080/00207411.2020.1717054

Cuijpers, P. (2017). Four decades of outcome research on psychotherapies for adult depression: An overview of a series of meta-analyses. *Canadian Psychology*, *58*(1), 7–19. https://doi.org/10.1037/cap0000096

Cuijpers, P. (2019). Targets and outcomes of psychotherapies for mental disorders: An overview. *World Psychiatry*, *18*(3), 276–285. https://doi.org/10.1002/wps.20661

Cuijpers, P., Noma, H., Karyotaki, E., Vinkers, C. H., Cipriani, A., & Furukawa, T. A. (2020). A network meta-analysis of the effects of psychotherapies, pharmacotherapies and their combination in the treatment of adult depression. *World Psychiatry*, *19*(1), 92–107. https://doi.org/10.1002/wps.20701

Davidson, L., Rowe, M., DiLeo, P., Bellamy, C., & Delphin-Rittmon, M. (2021). Recovery-oriented systems of care: A perspective on the past, present, and future. *Alcohol Research*, *41*(1), Article 09. https://doi.org/10.35946/arcr.v41.1.09

Davidson, L., Schmutte, T., Dinzeo, T., & Andres-Hyman, R. (2008). Remission and recovery in schizophrenia: Practitioner and patient perspectives. *Schizophrenia Bulletin*, *34*(1), 5–8. https://doi.org/10.1093/schbul/sbm122

Decker, S. E., Kiluk, B. D., Frankforter, T., Babuscio, T., Nich, C., & Carroll, K. M. (2016). Just showing up is not enough: Homework adherence and outcome in cognitive-behavioral therapy for cocaine dependence. *Journal of Consulting and Clinical Psychology*, *84*(10), 907–912. https://doi.org/10.1037/ccp0000126

Drake, R. E., Deegan, P. E., & Rapp, C. (2010). The promise of shared decision making in mental health. *Psychiatric Rehabilitation Journal*, *34*(1), 7–13. https://doi.org/10.2975/34.1.2010.7.13

Elwyn, G., Edwards, A., & Thompson, R. (Eds.). (2016). *Shared decision making in health care: Achieving evidence-based patient choice* (3rd ed.). Oxford University Press. https://doi.org/10.1093/acprof:oso/9780198723448.001.0001

Enriquez, J. (2019). *State involuntary commitment statutes: How can policy reflect patient-centered care* [Master's thesis, University of Pittsburgh]. D-Scholarship @ Pitt. https://d-scholarship.pitt.edu/36882/

Escobedo, P., Allem, J. P., Baezconde-Garbanati, L., & Unger, J. B. (2018). Cultural values associated with substance use among Hispanic emerging adults in Southern California. *Addictive Behaviors*, *77*, 267–271. https://doi.org/10.1016/j.addbeh.2017.07.018

Fahey, T. D., Insel, P. M., Roth, W. T., & Insel, C. (2018). *Fit & well: Core concepts and labs in physical fitness and wellness* (13th ed.). McGraw-Hill Education.

Fernández, D., Vigo, D., Sampson, N. A., Hwang, I., Aguilar-Gaxiola, S., Al-Hamzawi, A. O., Alonso, J., Andrade, L. H., Bromet, E. J., de Girolamo, G., de Jonge, P.,

Florescu, S., Gureje, O., Hinkov, H., Hu, C., Karam, E. G., Karam, G., Kawakami, N., Kiejna, A., . . . Haro, J. M. (2021). Patterns of care and dropout rates from outpatient mental healthcare in low-, middle- and high-income countries from the World Health Organization's World Mental Health Survey Initiative. *Psychological Medicine, 51*(12), 2104–2116. https://doi.org/10.1017/S0033291720000884

Fernandez, E., Salem, D., Swift, J. K., & Ramtahal, N. (2015). Meta-analysis of dropout from cognitive behavioral therapy: Magnitude, timing, and moderators. *Journal of Consulting and Clinical Psychology, 83*(6), 1108–1122. https://doi.org/10.1037/ccp0000044

Fonagy, P., & Luyten, P. (2019). Fidelity vs. flexibility in the implementation of psychotherapies: Time to move on. *World Psychiatry, 18*(3), 270–271. https://doi.org/10.1002/wps.20657

Fox, J. C., & Lipstein, E. A. (2020). Shared decision making in gastroenterology: Challenges and opportunities. *Mayo Clinic Proceedings: Innovations, Quality & Outcomes, 4*(2), 183–189. https://doi.org/10.1016/j.mayocpiqo.2019.11.003

Friedrichs, A., Spies, M., Härter, M., & Buchholz, A. (2016). Patient preferences and shared decision making in the treatment of substance use disorders: A systematic review of the literature. *PLOS ONE, 11*(1), Article e0145817. https://doi.org/10.1371/journal.pone.0145817

Gambino, M., Pavlo, A., & Ross, D. A. (2016). Recovery in mind: Perspectives from postgraduate psychiatric trainees. *Academic Psychiatry, 40*(3), 481–488. https://doi.org/10.1007/s40596-015-0414-x

Gao, S., Corrigan, P. W., Qin, S., & Nieweglowski, K. (2019). Comparing Chinese and European American mental health decision making. *Journal of Mental Health, 28*(2), 141–147. https://doi.org/10.1080/09638237.2017.1417543

Gill, H. S. (1988). Working through resistances of intrapsychic and environmental origin. *The International Journal of Psycho-Analysis, 69*(Pt. 4), 535–550.

Gill, K. J. (2006). With recovery now in our public policy, is recovery in danger? *Psychiatric Rehabilitation Journal, 30*(1), 7–8. https://doi.org/10.2975/30.2006.7.8

Girard, J. M., Wright, A. G. C., Beeney, J. E., Lazarus, S. A., Scott, L. N., Stepp, S. D., & Pilkonis, P. A. (2017). Interpersonal problems across levels of the psychopathology hierarchy. *Comprehensive Psychiatry, 79*, 53–69. https://doi.org/10.1016/j.comppsych.2017.06.014

Green-Hennessy, S. (2018). Suspension of the National Registry of Evidence-Based Programs and Practices: The importance of adhering to the evidence. *Substance Abuse Treatment, Prevention, and Policy, 13*(1), Article 26. https://doi.org/10.1186/s13011-018-0162-5

Hacker, K., Arsenault, L., Franco, I., Shaligram, D., Sidor, M., Olfson, M., & Goldstein, J. (2014). Referral and follow-up after mental health screening in commercially insured adolescents. *The Journal of Adolescent Health, 55*(1), 17–23. https://doi.org/10.1016/j.jadohealth.2013.12.012

Hajizadeh, N., Uhler, L. M., & Pérez Figueroa, R. E. (2015). Understanding patients' and doctors' attitudes about shared decision making for advance care planning. *Health Expectations, 18*(6), 2054–2065. https://doi.org/10.1111/hex.12285

Herrera, D. J., van de Veerdonk, W., Berhe, N. M., Talboom, S., van Loo, M., Alejos, A. R., Ferrari, A., & Van Hal, G. (2023). Mixed-method systematic review and meta-analysis of shared decision-making tools for cancer screening. *Cancers, 15*(15), Article 3867. https://doi.org/10.3390/cancers15153867

Himmerich, H., & Hamilton, A. (2022). Mood stabilizers: Side effects, contraindications, and interactions. In P. Riederer, G. Laux, T. Nagatsu, W. Le, & C. Riederer (Eds.), *NeuroPsychopharmacotherapy* (pp. 1447–1467). Springer. https://doi.org/10.1007/978-3-030-62059-2_40

Hogan, M. F. (2003). The President's New Freedom Commission: Recommendations to transform mental health care in America. *Psychiatric Services, 54*(11), 1467–1474. https://doi.org/10.1176/appi.ps.54.11.1467

Hornik-Lurie, T., Shalev, A., Haknazar, L., Garber Epstein, P., Ziedenberg-Rehav, L., & Moran, G. S. (2018). Implementing recovery-oriented interventions with staff in a psychiatric hospital: A mixed-methods study. *Journal of Psychiatric and Mental Health Nursing, 25*(9–10), 569–581. https://doi.org/10.1111/jpm.12502

Horst, P. T., Spreen, M., de Vries, E., & Bogaerts, S. (2023). Facilitating shared decision making in forensic psychiatry: The HKT-R Spider app. *Journal of Forensic Psychology Research and Practice, 23*(3), 328–343. https://doi.org/10.1080/24732850.2022.2028394

Huang, X., Harris, L. M., Funsch, K. M., Fox, K. R., & Ribeiro, J. D. (2022). Efficacy of psychotropic medications on suicide and self-injury: A meta-analysis of randomized controlled trials. *Translational Psychiatry, 12*(1), Article 400. https://doi.org/10.1038/s41398-022-02173-9

Ipsen, C., & Goe, R. (2016). Factors associated with consumer engagement and satisfaction with the Vocational Rehabilitation program. *Journal of Vocational Rehabilitation, 44*(1), 85–96. https://doi.org/10.3233/JVR-150782

Isohanni, M., Jääskeläinen, E., Miller, B. J., Hulkko, A., Tiihonen, J., Möller, H.-J., Hartikainen, S., Huhtaniska, S., & Lieslehto, J. (2021). Medication management of antipsychotic treatment in schizophrenia—A narrative review. *Human Psychopharmacology, 36*(2), Article e2765. https://doi.org/10.1002/hup.2765

Iyengar, S. S., & Lepper, M. R. (1999). Rethinking the value of choice: A cultural perspective on intrinsic motivation. *Journal of Personality and Social Psychology, 76*(3), 349–366. https://doi.org/10.1037/0022-3514.76.3.349

Jacobson, N., & Curtis, L. (2000). Recovery as policy in mental health services: Strategies emerging from the states. *Psychiatric Rehabilitation Journal, 23*(4), 333–341. https://doi.org/10.1037/h0095146

Jonas, E., Graupmann, V., Kayser, D. N., Zanna, M., Traut-Mattausch, E., & Frey, D. (2009). Culture, self, and the emergence of reactance: Is there a "universal" freedom? *Journal of Experimental Social Psychology, 45*(5), 1068–1080. https://doi.org/10.1016/j.jesp.2009.06.005

Kaduszkiewicz, H., Bochon, B., van den Bussche, H., Hansmann-Wiest, J., & van der Leeden, C. (2017). The medical treatment of homeless people. *Deutsches Ärzteblatt International, 114*(40), 673–679. https://doi.org/10.3238/arztebl.2017.0673

Kazantzis, N., Whittington, C., Zelencich, L., Kyrios, M., Norton, P. J., & Hofmann, S. G. (2016). Quantity and quality of homework compliance: A meta-analysis of relations with outcome in cognitive behavior therapy. *Behavior Therapy, 47*(5), 755–772. https://doi.org/10.1016/j.beth.2016.05.002

Kirmayer, L. J., & Minas, H. (2008). The future of cultural psychiatry: An international perspective. In C. G. Helman (Ed.), *Medical anthropology* (pp. 438–446). Routledge.

Kraepelin, E. (1919). *Dementia praecox and paraphrenia* (R. M. Barclay, Trans.; G. M. Robertson, Ed.). E. & S. Livingstone.

Krupnik, V. (2023). The therapeutic alliance as active inference: The role of trust and self-efficacy. *Journal of Contemporary Psychotherapy, 53*(3), 207–215. https://doi.org/10.1007/s10879-022-09576-1

Lappan, S. N., Brown, A. W., & Hendricks, P. S. (2020). Dropout rates of in-person psychosocial substance use disorder treatments: A systematic review and meta-analysis. *Addiction, 115*(2), 201–207. https://doi.org/10.1111/add.14793

Lee, E. J., Lam, C., & Ditchman, N. (2015). Self-determination and cultural considerations: An Asian perspective. In P. W. Corrigan (Ed.), *Person-centered care for mental illness: The evolution of adherence and self-determination* (pp. 211–234). American Psychological Association. https://doi.org/10.1037/14644-012

Leeuwerik, T., Cavanagh, K., & Strauss, C. (2019). Patient adherence to cognitive behavioural therapy for obsessive-compulsive disorder: A systematic review and meta-analysis. *Journal of Anxiety Disorders, 68*, Article 102135. https://doi.org/10.1016/j.janxdis.2019.102135

Lemstra, M., Bird, Y., Nwankwo, C., Rogers, M., & Moraros, J. (2016). Weight loss intervention adherence and factors promoting adherence: A meta-analysis. *Patient Preference and Adherence, 10*, 1547–1559. https://doi.org/10.2147/PPA.S103649

Leonhardt, B. L., Huling, K., Hamm, J. A., Roe, D., Hasson-Ohayon, I., McLeod, H. J., & Lysaker, P. H. (2017). Recovery and serious mental illness: A review of current clinical and research paradigms and future directions. *Expert Review of Neurotherapeutics, 17*(11), 1117–1130. https://doi.org/10.1080/14737175.2017.1378099

Levengood, T. W., Yoon, G. H., Davoust, M. J., Ogden, S. N., Marshall, B. D. L., Cahill, S. R., & Bazzi, A. R. (2021). Supervised injection facilities as harm reduction: A systematic review. *American Journal of Preventive Medicine, 61*(5), 738–749. https://doi.org/10.1016/j.amepre.2021.04.017

Liberman, R. P. (2008). *Recovery from disability: Manual of psychiatric rehabilitation.* American Psychiatric Publishing.

Linden, M. (2017). Definition and assessment of disability in mental disorders under the perspective of the International Classification of Functioning Disability and Health (ICF). *Behavioral Sciences & the Law, 35*(2), 124–134. https://doi.org/10.1002/bsl.2283

Lönnqvist, J. (1985). Evaluation of psychosocial treatments. *Acta Psychiatrica Scandinavica, 371*, 141–150. https://doi.org/10.1111/j.1600-0447.1985.tb08530.x

Mandal, R., & Ose, S. O. (2020). Managing absence and dropout in vocational rehabilitation—A mixed-methods analysis of practices and perspectives among vocational rehabilitation companies in Norway. *Disability and Rehabilitation, 42*(17), 2471–2481. https://doi.org/10.1080/09638288.2018.1561957

Mantzouranis, G., Baier, V., Holzer, L., Urben, S., & Villard, E. (2019). Clinical significance of assertive community treatment among adolescents. *Social Psychiatry and Psychiatric Epidemiology, 54*(4), 445–453. https://doi.org/10.1007/s00127-018-1613-z

Marchand, K., Beaumont, S., Westfall, J., MacDonald, S., Harrison, S., Marsh, D. C., Schechter, M. T., & Oviedo-Joekes, E. (2019). Conceptualizing patient-centered care for substance use disorder treatment: Findings from a systematic scoping review. *Substance Abuse Treatment, Prevention, and Policy, 14*(1), Article 37. https://doi.org/10.1186/s13011-019-0227-0

Martínez-González, N. A., Neuner-Jehle, S., Plate, A., Rosemann, T., & Senn, O. (2018). Correction to: The effects of shared decision-making compared to usual care for prostate cancer screening decisions: A systematic review and meta-analysis. *BMC Cancer, 18*(1), 1196. https://doi.org/10.1186/s12885-018-4794-7

Matweychuk, W., DiGiuseppe, R., & Gulyayeva, O. (2019). A Comparison of REBT with other cognitive behavior therapies. In M. E. Bernard & W. Dryden (Eds.), *Advances in REBT: Theory, practice, research, measurement, prevention and promotion* (pp. 47–77). Springer. https://doi.org/10.1007/978-3-319-93118-0_3

Messer, S. B. (2002). A psychodynamic perspective on resistance in psychotherapy: Vive la resistance [Long live the resistance]. *Journal of Clinical Psychology, 58*(2), 157–163. https://doi.org/10.1002/jclp.1139

Miglietta, E., Belessiotis-Richards, C., Ruggeri, M., & Priebe, S. (2018). Scales for assessing patient satisfaction with mental health care: A systematic review. *Journal of Psychiatric Research, 100*, 33–46. https://doi.org/10.1016/j.jpsychires.2018.02.014

Miller, C. H., & Quick, B. L. (2010). Sensation seeking and psychological reactance as health risk predictors for an emerging adult population. *Health Communication, 25*(3), 266–275. https://doi.org/10.1080/10410231003698945

Miller, W. R., & Rose, G. S. (2010). Motivational interviewing in relational context. *American Psychologist, 65*(4), 298–299. https://doi.org/10.1037/a0019487

Mitropoulou, P., Grüner-Hegge, N., Reinhold, J., & Papadopoulou, C. (2023). Shared decision making in cardiology: A systematic review and meta-analysis. *Heart, 109*(1), 34–39. https://doi.org/10.1136/heartjnl-2022-321050

Munthe, C., Sandman, L., Nykänen, P., & El Alti, L. (2016, August 17–20). *Person centredness and shared decision-making in forensic care, social services and public health* [Paper presentation]. 30th European Conference of the Philosophy of Medicine and Healthcare, Zagreb, Croatia.

Naslund, J. A., Aschbrenner, K. A., Marsch, L. A., & Bartels, S. J. (2016). The future of mental health care: Peer-to-peer support and social media. *Epidemiology and Psychiatric Sciences, 25*(2), 113–122. https://doi.org/10.1017/S2045796015001067

Neiman, A. B., Ruppar, T., Ho, M., Garber, L., Weidle, P. J., Hong, Y., George, M. G., & Thorpe, P. G. (2017). CDC grand rounds: Improving medication adherence for chronic disease management—Innovations and opportunities. *Morbidity and Mortality Weekly Report, 66*(45), 1248–1251. https://doi.org/10.15585/mmwr.mm6645a2

New Freedom Commission on Mental Health. (2003). *Achieving the promise: Transforming mental health care in America: Final report* (DHHS Publication No. SMA-03-3832). U.S. Department of Health and Human Services. https://govinfo.library.unt.edu/mentalhealthcommission/reports/FinalReport/downloads/FinalReport.pdf

Ngu, H., Neo, S. H., Koh, E. Y. L., Ho, H., & Tan, N. C. (2022). Making shared decisions with older men selecting treatment for lower urinary tract symptoms secondary to benign prostatic hyperplasia (LUTS/BPH): A pilot randomized trial. *Journal of Patient-Reported Outcomes, 6*(1), Article 112. https://doi.org/10.1186/s41687-022-00519-x

Norcross, J. C., & Wampold, B. E. (2019). *Psychotherapy relationships that work: Evidence-based therapist responsiveness* (3rd ed.). Oxford University Press.

Okasha, A., Arboleda-Florez, J., & Sartorius, N. (Eds.). (2008). *Ethics, culture, and psychiatry: International perspectives*. American Psychiatric Association Publishing.

Okkels, N., Kristiansen, C. B., Munk-Jørgensen, P., & Sartorius, N. (2018). Urban mental health: Challenges and perspectives. *Current Opinion in Psychiatry, 31*(3), 258–264. https://doi.org/10.1097/YCO.0000000000000413

O'Leary, C., Ralphs, R., Stevenson, J., Smith, A., Harrison, J., Kiss, Z., & Armitage, H. (2024). The effectiveness of abstinence-based and harm reduction-based interventions in reducing problematic substance use in adults who are experiencing homelessness in high income countries: A systematic review and meta-analysis: A systematic review. *Campbell Systematic Reviews, 20*(2), Article e1396. https://doi.org/10.1002/cl2.1396

Pace, B. T., Dembe, A., Soma, C. S., Baldwin, S. A., Atkins, D. C., & Imel, Z. E. (2017). A multivariate meta-analysis of motivational interviewing process and outcome. *Psychology of Addictive Behaviors, 31*(5), 524–533. https://doi.org/10.1037/adb0000280

Pilgrim, D. (2008). "Recovery" and current mental health policy. *Chronic Illness, 4*(4), 295–304. https://doi.org/10.1177/1742395308097863

Price-Robertson, R., Obradovic, A., & Morgan, B. (2017). Relational recovery: Beyond individualism in the recovery approach. *Advances in Mental Health, 15*(2), 108–120. https://doi.org/10.1080/18387357.2016.1243014

Prowse, P.-T., Nagel, T., Meadows, G. N., & Enticott, J. C. (2015). Treatment fidelity over the last decade in psychosocial clinical trials outcome studies: A systematic review. *African Journal of Psychiatry, 18*(2), 1–8. https://doi.org/10.4172/Psychiatry.1000258

Qin, D. B., & Chang, T.-F. (2012). Asian American fathers. In N. J. Cabrera & C. S. Tamis-LeMonda (Eds.), *Handbook of father involvement: Multidisciplinary perspectives* (2nd ed., pp. 261–278). Routledge.

Quick, B. L., & Stephenson, M. T. (2008). Examining the role of trait reactance and sensation seeking on perceived threat, state reactance, and reactance restoration. *Human Communication Research, 34*(3), 448–476. https://doi.org/10.1111/j.1468-2958.2008.00328.x

Redlich, A. D., Steadman, H. J., Robbins, P. C., & Swanson, J. W. (2006). Use of the criminal justice system to leverage mental health treatment: Effects on treatment adherence and satisfaction. *The Journal of the American Academy of Psychiatry and the Law, 34*(3), 292–299.

Reser, M. P., Slikboer, R., & Rossell, S. L. (2019). A systematic review of factors that influence the efficacy of cognitive remediation therapy in schizophrenia. *The Australian and New Zealand Journal of Psychiatry, 53*(7), 624–641. https://doi.org/10.1177/0004867419853348

Richter, D., & Hoffmann, H. (2019). Effectiveness of supported employment in non-trial routine implementation: Systematic review and meta-analysis. *Social Psychiatry and Psychiatric Epidemiology, 54*(5), 525–531. https://doi.org/10.1007/s00127-018-1577-z

Rogers, E. S., Chamberlin, J., Ellison, M. L., & Crean, T. (1997). A consumer-constructed scale to measure empowerment among users of mental health services. *Psychiatric Services, 48*(8), 1042–1047. https://doi.org/10.1176/ps.48.8.1042

Rogers, E. S., Ralph, R. O., & Salzer, M. S. (2010). Validating the empowerment scale with a multisite sample of consumers of mental health services. *Psychiatric Services, 61*(9), 933–936. https://doi.org/10.1176/ps.2010.61.9.933

Rudnick, A. (2008a). Ethical implications of emotional impairment. In L. C. Charland & P. Zachar (Eds.), *Fact and value in emotion* (pp. 87–99). John Benjamins Publishing. https://doi.org/10.1075/ceb.4.06rud

Rudnick, A. (2008b). Recovery from schizophrenia: A philosophical framework. *American Journal of Psychiatric Rehabilitation, 11*(3), 267–278. https://doi.org/10.1080/15487760802186360

Ruiz-Pérez, I., Bermúdez-Tamayo, C., & Rodríguez-Barranco, M. (2017). Socioeconomic factors linked with mental health during the recession: A multilevel analysis. *International Journal for Equity in Health, 16*(1), Article 45. https://doi.org/10.1186/s12939-017-0518-x

Semahegn, A., Torpey, K., Manu, A., Assefa, N., Tesfaye, G., & Ankomah, A. (2020). Psychotropic medication non-adherence and its associated factors among patients with major psychiatric disorders: A systematic review and meta-analysis. *Systematic Reviews, 9*(1), Article 17. https://doi.org/10.1186/s13643-020-1274-3

Seyedfatemi, N., Ahmadzad Asl, M., Bahrami, R., & Haghani, H. (2021). The effect of the virtual social network-based psycho-education on the hope of family caregivers of clients with severe mental disorders. *Archives of Psychiatric Nursing, 35*(3), 290–295. https://doi.org/10.1016/j.apnu.2021.02.004

Shay, L. A., & Lafata, J. E. (2015). Where is the evidence? A systematic review of shared decision making and patient outcomes. *Medical Decision Making, 35*(1), 114–131. https://doi.org/10.1177/0272989X14551638

Shin, S., & Choi, H. (2020). A systematic review on peer support services related to the mental health services utilization for people with severe mental illness. *Journal of Korean Academy of Psychiatric and Mental Health Nursing, 29*(1), 51–63. https://doi.org/10.12934/jkpmhn.2020.29.1.51

Shorey, S., & Chua, J. Y. X. (2023). Effectiveness of peer support interventions for adults with depressive symptoms: A systematic review and meta-analysis. *Journal of Mental Health, 32*(2), 465–479. https://doi.org/10.1080/09638237.2021.2022630

Siegel, J. T., Lienemann, B. A., & Rosenberg, B. D. (2017). Resistance, reactance, and misinterpretation: Highlighting the challenge of persuading people with depression to seek help. *Social and Personality Psychology Compass, 11*(6), Article e12322. https://doi.org/10.1111/spc3.12322

Slade, M. (2009). *Personal recovery and mental illness: A guide for mental health professionals.* Cambridge University Press. https://doi.org/10.1017/CBO9780511581649

Slade, M. (2017). Implementing shared decision making in routine mental health care. *World Psychiatry, 16*(2), 146–153. https://doi.org/10.1002/wps.20412

Slade, M., & Longden, E. (2015). Empirical evidence about recovery and mental health. *BMC Psychiatry, 15*(1), Article 285. https://doi.org/10.1186/s12888-015-0678-4

Song, K., & Wu, D. (2022). Shared decision-making in the management of patients with inflammatory bowel disease. *World Journal of Gastroenterology, 28*(26), 3092–3100. https://doi.org/10.3748/wjg.v28.i26.3092

Speed, B. C., Goldstein, B. L., & Goldfried, M. R. (2018). Assertiveness training: A forgotten evidence-based treatment. *Clinical Psychology: Science and Practice, 25*(1). https://doi.org/10.1111/cpsp.12216

Sprague, J., & Hayes, J. (2000). Self-determination and empowerment: A feminist standpoint analysis of talk about disability. *American Journal of Community Psychology, 28*(5), 671–695. https://doi.org/10.1023/A:1005197704441

Stivers, T., & Timmermans, S. (2020). Medical authority under siege: How clinicians transform patient resistance into acceptance. *Journal of Health and Social Behavior, 61*(1), 60–78. https://doi.org/10.1177/0022146520902740

Substance Abuse and Mental Health Services Administration. (2023a). *Evidence-Based Practices Resource Center*. https://www.samhsa.gov/resource-search/ebp

Substance Abuse and Mental Health Services Administration. (2023b). *Key substance use and mental health indicators in the United States: Results from the 2022 National Survey on Drug Use and Health* (HHS Publication No. PEP23-07-01-006, NSDUH Series H-58). Center for Behavioral Health Statistics and Quality, Substance Abuse and Mental Health Services Administration. https://www.samhsa.gov/data/sites/default/files/reports/rpt42731/2022-nsduh-nnr.pdf

Sweeney, A., Gillard, S., Wykes, T., & Rose, D. (2015). The role of fear in mental health service users' experiences: A qualitative exploration. *Social Psychiatry and Psychiatric Epidemiology, 50*(7), 1079–1087. https://doi.org/10.1007/s00127-015-1028-z

Szasz, T. (2007). *Coercion as cure: A critical history of psychiatry*. Transaction Publishers.

Tang, W., & Kreindler, D. (2017). Supporting homework compliance in cognitive behavioural therapy: Essential features of mobile apps. *JMIR Mental Health, 4*(2), Article e20. https://doi.org/10.2196/mental.5283

Thomas, E. C., Ben-David, S., Treichler, E., Roth, S., Dixon, L. B., Salzer, M., & Zisman-Ilani, Y. (2021). A systematic review of shared decision-making interventions for service users with serious mental illnesses: State of the science and future directions. *Psychiatric Services, 72*(11), 1288–1300. https://doi.org/10.1176/appi.ps.202000429

Thornicroft, G. (2020). People with severe mental illness as the perpetrators and victims of violence: Time for a new public health approach. *The Lancet Public Health, 5*(2), e72–e73. https://doi.org/10.1016/S2468-2667(20)30002-5

Thornicroft, G., Deb, T., & Henderson, C. (2016). Community mental health care worldwide: Current status and further developments. *World Psychiatry, 15*(3), 276–286. https://doi.org/10.1002/wps.20349

Thornicroft, G., & Henderson, C. (2016). Joint decision making and reduced need for compulsory psychiatric admission. *JAMA Psychiatry, 73*(7), 647–648. https://doi.org/10.1001/jamapsychiatry.2016.0571

Tse, S., Tsoi, E. W., Hamilton, B., O'Hagan, M., Shepherd, G., Slade, M., Whitley, R., & Petrakis, M. (2016). Uses of strength-based interventions for people with serious mental illness: A critical review. *The International Journal of Social Psychiatry, 62*(3), 281–291. https://doi.org/10.1177/0020764015623970

Upshur, C. C., Jenkins, D., Weinreb, L., Gelberg, L., & Orvek, E. A. (2018). Homeless women's service use, barriers, and motivation for participating in substance use treatment. *The American Journal of Drug and Alcohol Abuse, 44*(2), 252–262. https://doi.org/10.1080/00952990.2017.1357183

Van Dorn, R., Volavka, J., & Johnson, N. (2012). Mental disorder and violence: Is there a relationship beyond substance use? *Social Psychiatry and Psychiatric Epidemiology, 47*, 487–503. https://doi.org/10.1007/s00127-011-0356-x

van Nistelrooij, I., Visse, M., Spekkink, A., & de Lange, J. (2017). How shared is shared decision-making? A care-ethical view on the role of partner and family. *Journal of Medical Ethics, 43*(9), 637–644. https://doi.org/10.1136/medethics-2016-103791

Velligan, D. I., Li, F., Sebastian, V., Kennedy, C., & Mintz, J. (2023). A pilot study examining feasibility and initial efficacy of remotely delivered cognitive adaptation training. *Schizophrenia Bulletin Open*, *4*(1), Article sgad028. https://doi.org/10.1093/schizbullopen/sgad028

Velligan, D. I., Tai, S., Roberts, D. L., Maples-Aguilar, N., Brown, M., Mintz, J., & Turkington, D. (2015). A randomized controlled trial comparing cognitive behavior therapy, cognitive adaptation training, their combination and treatment as usual in chronic schizophrenia. *Schizophrenia Bulletin*, *41*(3), 597–603. https://doi.org/10.1093/schbul/sbu127

Velligan, D. I., Weiden, P. J., Sajatovic, M., Scott, J., Carpenter, D., Ross, R., & Docherty, J. P. (2010). Assessment of adherence problems in patients with serious and persistent mental illness: Recommendations from the *Expert Consensus Guidelines*. *Journal of Psychiatric Practice*, *16*(1), 34–45. https://doi.org/10.1097/01.pra.0000367776.96012.ca

Vuckovich, P. K. (2010). Compliance versus adherence in serious and persistent mental illness. *Nursing Ethics*, *17*(1), 77–85. https://doi.org/10.1177/0969733009352047

Wade, D. T., & Halligan, P. W. (2017). The biopsychosocial model of illness: A model whose time has come. *Clinical Rehabilitation*, *31*(8), 995–1004. https://doi.org/10.1177/0269215517709890

Walker, E. R., Cummings, J. R., Hockenberry, J. M., & Druss, B. G. (2015). Insurance status, use of mental health services, and unmet need for mental health care in the United States. *Psychiatric Services*, *66*(6), 578–584. https://doi.org/10.1176/appi.ps.201400248

Wang, S.-M., Han, C., Bahk, W.-M., Lee, S.-J., Patkar, A. A., Masand, P. S., & Pae, C.-U. (2018). Addressing the side effects of contemporary antidepressant drugs: A comprehensive review. *Chonnam Medical Journal*, *54*(2), 101–112. https://doi.org/10.4068/cmj.2018.54.2.101

White, S., Foster, R., Marks, J., Morshead, R., Goldsmith, L., Barlow, S., Sin, J., & Gillard, S. (2020). The effectiveness of one-to-one peer support in mental health services: A systematic review and meta-analysis. *BMC Psychiatry*, *20*(1), Article 534. https://doi.org/10.1186/s12888-020-02923-3

World Health Organization. (2021). *Suicide worldwide in 2019: Global health estimates*. https://iris.who.int/bitstream/handle/10665/341728/9789240026643-eng.pdf?sequence=1

Zimmerman, M., Morgan, T. A., & Stanton, K. (2018). The severity of psychiatric disorders. *World Psychiatry*, *17*(3), 258–275. https://doi.org/10.1002/wps.20569

Zisman-Ilani, Y., Roth, R. M., & Mistler, L. A. (2021). Time to support extensive implementation of shared decision making in psychiatry. *JAMA Psychiatry*, *78*(11), 1183–1184. https://doi.org/10.1001/jamapsychiatry.2021.2247

2 THE "RATIONAL" DECISION MAKER

SARAH E. COATES AND PATRICK W. CORRIGAN

One way behavioral scientists have made sense of shared decision making (SDM) is by positing people as rational actors making decisions about their health and wellness options. Rational patients might be viewed as coolly and solely weighing costs and benefits in a prior and planful manner. SDM helps the person with the rational process; however, as we propose and review in this chapter. the model has limits: Although it seems that rational patients make "conscious" comparisons of the advantages and disadvantages of treatment decisions, many real-life decisions are influenced and made implicitly and outside of awareness. Rather than planning with foresight, treatment decisions and behaviors are influenced by immediate exigencies. It is not the consideration on Monday that leads to whether the person takes medication Thursday afternoon but, rather, the effect of more salient issues on Thursday morning. The idea of the rational patient suggests cold and calculated decisions when, indeed, many of these are emotional enterprises.

We review each of these limitations by summarizing evidence that expands the narrow assertion about the rational patient into more complex behavior representing the multifaceted experience of health decision making. We begin with a case example (see Exhibit 2.1) that is referenced throughout

https://doi.org/10.1037/0000478-002
Shared Decision Making and Serious Mental Illness, P. W. Corrigan (Editor)

EXHIBIT 2.1. Case Example: Sylvia

Sylvia is a 48-year-old Black woman who has been diagnosed with recurrent major depressive disorder over the past 20 years. She meets criteria of experiencing depressed mood, decreased interest in engaging in activities, fatigue, feelings of worthlessness, and recurrent thoughts of death that she's had for the past 4 weeks. She has had multiple hospital admissions resulting from episodes of severe depression as well as instances of suicidal ideation. Sylvia has been living with her husband for the past 5 years and was fired 3 weeks ago from her job of 2 years. She has been admitted to inpatient hospitalization because of a recent instance of active suicidal ideation with plan and intent. Before her current admission, Sylvia was hospitalized three times because of suicidal ideation.

After a 7-day intensive inpatient stay, Sylvia has been cleared to be discharged back home to live with her husband. She now feels uncertain about how to proceed moving forward and needs help making decisions regarding how to navigate employment options. Sylvia is nervous about starting the process and concerned about how she will perform in a new job. She sits down with a health care provider to go through the shared decision making process. With the help of her health care provider, Sylvia has identified as her goal finding a new job after her discharge. To help her achieve this goal, Sylvia's provider informs her that she has the following three options: (a) She can meet with a job coach, (b) she can be connected with a peer support person, or (c) she can pursue additional schooling.

Note. Case examples in this book are hypothetical.

the chapter to highlight the rational process in SDM as well as limitations to the model. We then summarize rational actor models that describe health decision making and contrast them with behavioral economics and other sociological critiques. After that is a section organized in terms of three limitations to the rational patient model. We end by considering what these alternatives mean for the ongoing study of SDM in health decisions and behaviors. Although we acknowledge that various models explaining decision-making processes exist, we chose to focus the scope of this chapter on the rational patient model.

One way to expand discussions on SDM is to recognize it as one example of the broader set of decisions and behaviors related to a person's pursuit of health. Health decisions involve both a choice ("Yes, I will meet with my job coach today") and a behavior (the person and job coach come together at a prospective job site). Hence, research and theory focus not only on whether people are doing what they should but also on the various processes that affect independent decision making and behaviors related to health, thus broadening the discussion to include the insights of psychological models related to decision making. Still, within these models, the link between decisions and behaviors is not easily explained. There is continued debate about the primacy of the two phenomena—decisions lead to behaviors, or behavior change causes corresponding decisions to change—versus a perspective that linking the two may be extraneous to important behavioral science goals altogether.

MODELS OF RATIONAL PATIENTS

Figure 2.1 summarizes models that explain health decision making. We have divided models into those that have evolved out of psychology—the mostly cognitive processes of the individual—and those of sociology, resting decision processes on the social interactions in which they occur.

Psychological Models

Several theories have been well tested to explain health decisions as a rational process, one in which a person makes health decisions based on the balance

FIGURE 2.1. Models That Explain the Rational Decision Maker in the World From a Psychological and a Sociological Perspective

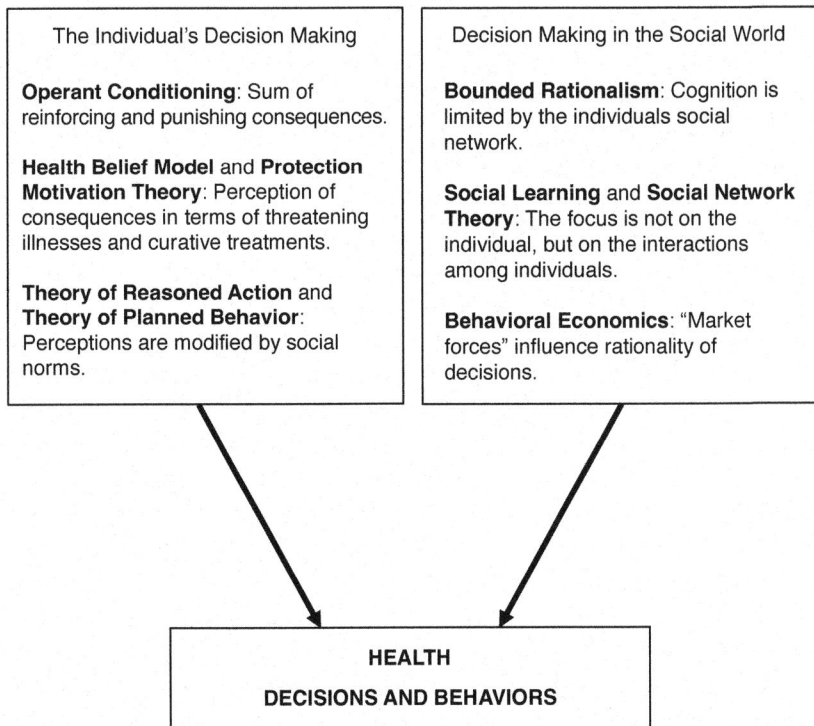

The Individual's Decision Making	Decision Making in the Social World
Operant Conditioning: Sum of reinforcing and punishing consequences.	**Bounded Rationalism**: Cognition is limited by the individuals social network.
Health Belief Model and **Protection Motivation Theory**: Perception of consequences in terms of threatening illnesses and curative treatments.	**Social Learning** and **Social Network Theory**: The focus is not on the individual, but on the interactions among individuals.
Theory of Reasoned Action and **Theory of Planned Behavior**: Perceptions are modified by social norms.	**Behavioral Economics**: "Market forces" influence rationality of decisions.

HEALTH DECISIONS AND BEHAVIORS

of perceived costs and benefits. More than 50 years ago, the health belief model (HBM) was posed by health care providers and services researchers as a decisional process influenced by the harm of a clinical illness or condition (Champion & Skinner, 2008; Ragin et al., 2020; Rosenstock, 1966, 1974). *Clinical harm* was defined as perceived susceptibility (i.e., the likelihood that an individual will contract a condition) and perceived severity (i.e., the effect of a condition as measured by symptoms, quality of life, and disability) relating to an individual's perceived health outcome. Decisions based on susceptibility and severity are moderated by perceived benefits (e.g., Does changing the condition yield a positive advantage for the person?) and perceived barrier (e.g., Are there elements of changing the condition that seem harmful or prevent them from engaging in changing the condition?). Although the HBM has attracted careful and comprehensive critiques since its development (Stroebe & Stroebe, 1995), it continues to be incorporated into contemporary research in the field of health psychology and has been applied to a range of health behaviors (Taflinger & Sattler, 2024), including adherence behaviors (Jones et al., 2014), smoking risk behaviors (Mantler, 2013), mammography screenings (Ritchie et al., 2021), and physical activity (Plotnikoff et al., 2013).

Closely related to the HBM is protection motivation theory (PMT; Armitage & Conner, 2000; Rogers, 1983). In PMT, health behavior is framed as adaptive or maladaptive coping, which is determined by protection motivation. This kind of motivation is influenced by threat appraisals (based on perceived vulnerability and severity of illness) and coping appraisals (based on perceived efficacy of a behavior response).

Meta-analyses completed on the HBM (Harrison et al., 1992) and PMT (Floyd et al., 2000; Milne et al., 2000) yielded small to medium effect sizes in their explanations of health decisions. A recent meta-analysis examining the effectiveness of the HBM constructs (i.e., susceptibility, severity, benefits, and barriers) found variability regarding each construct's effectiveness as behavior change predictors; the perceived benefits and barriers produced a strong effect, perceived severity produced little effect, and perceived susceptibility produced a small insignificant effect (Carpenter, 2010).

The HBM and PMT reflect the more basic conceptualizations of operant and social learning theorists. Simply put, behaviors are driven by the effect of rewards and punishment (Skinner, 1953). In this light, environmental contingencies are expected to influence health behavior; people who have experienced the aversive events of an illness and positive interactions with a physician are likely to seek out that physician or similar doctors for future care. Classic operant theories have difficulty with "decision" as a research focus, instead believing only observable behaviors can be explained by psychological theory. More recent operant models, though, have sought to transcend limitations of an observable behavior by developing models of verbal learning, such as relational frame theory (Hayes et al., 2001), thus making significant contributions as demonstrated by increased publications in the field (Dymond et al., 2010; O'Connor et al., 2017; Raaymakers et al., 2019).

Bandura's (1977) social learning theory framed the effect of actual environmental contingencies as influenced by perceptions of, and expectations about, a behavior that evolve from previously experienced learning trials. It is not the assortment of past reinforcing and punishing consequences of a health behavior but, rather, how past learning has been experienced in the social world and the expectations those experiences engender. Bandura (1986) further elaborated on social learning effects by developing the idea of self-efficacy, a construct that fits prominently in the HBM and PMT (Conner & Norman, 2005; Glanz et al., 2008). *Self-efficacy* represents confidence in one's ability to carry out a specific behavior in a specific setting. Within the context of health decisions, findings from a meta-analysis demonstrating intervention-related changes in self-efficacy produced medium effects in intention and small to medium effects in health behavior change (Sheeran et al., 2016). The theory of reasoned action (TRA) seems to be a more direct social learning model relevant to understanding health decisions and behaviors (Ajzen & Fishbein, 1980; Fishbein & Ajzen, 1975). Similar to previous theories, the TRA proffers positive and negative evaluation of a behavior as central to moving ahead on said behavior. The theory also suggests perception of social norms to be an essential element of reasoned action; namely, recognition of an important other's preference vis-à-vis health behavior moderates the patient's decisions. Ajzen (1988) conceded that the TRA was limited to volitional behavior and developed the theory of planned behavior (TPB) by adding notions of perceived control. *Perceived control* represents actual management in a specific setting and a measure of confidence in one's ability in that setting (similar to self-efficacy). Findings from a meta-analysis of 237 prospective data sets of TRA and TPB, specifically reflecting health decisions, yielded medium to large effect sizes with intentions and attitudes emerging as important behavioral predictors (McEachan et al., 2011).

How is Sylvia's decision explained by the HBM? Sylvia, along with the help of her health care provider, considers the susceptibility and severity of her decision based on the perceived benefits and barriers of the options she has available. Through the SDM process of rationally weighing a variety of costs (e.g., financial costs, time requirements, and the process of applying to school) and benefits (e.g., immediate assistance in getting a job and therefore the ability to have money to pay her bills sooner) with her health care provider, Sylvia is able to identify the best possible solution is for her to meet with a job coach to help her find a new job. Based on this decision and with the support of her provider, Sylvia has scheduled a meeting with her job coach on Wednesday at 1 p.m. and is scheduled to be discharged tomorrow (Sunday). As a rational patient in the SDM process, Sylvia was able to identify goals for herself at this significant moment in her life, weigh the costs and benefits of a variety of options to help her achieve her goals, come to a decision based on the perceived benefits and barriers she identified with her health care provider, and create a plan for the next step in achieving her goals.

Sociological Models

Social learning theory represents a bridge to a broader sociological approach to decision making that explains help-seeking behavior beyond the individual's rational processes (Friedman & Hechter, 1988; Lindenberg, 1985). Sociological models reflect bounded rationality (Simon, 1955); namely, the power of individual cognition is limited by the social network in which an individual lives, acts, and decides. In social network theory, attributes of individuals are less important than their relationships and ties with other actors within the network. The ties that connect multiple units represent the convergence of the various social contacts of the network. Social unit may differ for each person and can consist of an individual or, more broadly, family, clan, or communities. An axiom of the social network approach to understanding social interaction is that social phenomena should be primarily conceived and investigated through the properties of relations between and within units instead of the properties of these units themselves. Pescosolido (1992) used social network theory to counter ideas of the rational patient, placing health decisions within the network of social unit interactions. It is not the solo, planful consideration of contingencies that drive health decisions but, rather, the dynamic, often immediate, and sometimes "irrational" products of social networks from which health decisions and behaviors evolve.

Bounded rationalism was further developed by behavioral economists. Kahneman and Tversky (1979) qualified individual decision making in terms of classical economics. They argued that people often rely on cognitive shortcuts that may not be the most rational but serve the perceived needs of specific moments in economic spaces (Q. Liu et al., 2022; Volpp et al., 2010). For example, Kahneman and Tversky (1979) developed cognitive heuristics to show that decisions and corresponding behaviors often rest on rules of thumb rather than on rational logic. The availability heuristic—the notion that perceived truth reflects the simple exposure to a phenomenon (Tversky & Kahneman, 1973)—offers a compelling example: A person believes cigarette smoking is not health threatening because "my father smoked two packs a day for 50 years." A review of the research literature showed that much of the work on behavioral economics has attempted to explain health behavior at the policy level, such as understanding monetary and time costs (O'Donohue & Cucciare, 2005; Schwartz & Hursh, 2023). A growing amount of research has applied concepts of behavioral economics to the clinical level to assist in promoting change across a variety of health decisions (Bickel et al., 2016; Bickel & Vuchinich, 2000).

CRITIQUES OF RATIONAL PATIENT MODELS

Although social network models add much to understanding health decisions, a rational actor model continues to dominate because of the one-on-one nature of SDM. Hence, SDM processes are often saturated with weighing costs and benefits of specific decisions. In this light, it is important for SDM providers to understand three limitations of the rational patient model: (a) Many decisions are not conscious, (b) immediate processes are especially effective, and (c) cognitive processes are influenced by emotions.

Many Implicit Health Decisions

The rational patient in SDM is assumed to purposefully list the costs and benefits of an intervention strategy or behavior and then develop a plan accordingly. This process is completed in conjunction with a designated health care provider. Many decisions, however, are made outside of awareness. For example, individuals may automatically associate medication or any other treatment with costs irrespective of whether they deliberately endorse the proposition that the treatment is beneficial. Social psychological research has convincingly shown that implicit, automatically activated associations differ from deliberately endorsed propositions (Gawronski & Bodenhausen, 2006; Greenwald & Nosek, 2009). Implicit reactions are typically characterized by rapidity, spontaneity (lack of conscious intention), efficiency (minimal use of attentional resources), inevitability (lack of control over initial activation), and unawareness of triggering cues (Bargh, 1994; Gawronski & Bodenhausen, 2006). In this context, implicitness suggests that the concept of enhancing health behavior can automatically activate positive or negative attributes if those concepts are associated with one another in memory. Well-established reaction-time tasks, such as the Implicit Association Test (IAT; Greenwald et al., 1998), measure automatic associations between two concepts (e.g., "Medication" and "Good") and may index implicit attitudes toward treatments. Indirect measures of implicit reactions are less susceptible to strategic response distortions and self-presentational strategies; therefore, they are particularly helpful in work on health decisions in which patients may hesitate to openly and honestly endorse negative attitudes toward treatments.

In addition, implicit versus explicit responses may independently predict outcome variables. A meta-analysis found that both implicit and explicit responses effectively predicted behavior; explicit measures demonstrated higher effect size variability (Greenwald et al., 2009). Another recent meta-analysis on the IAT concluded that implicit reactions and explicit reactions provided unique contributions in predicting behavior; implicit measures were associated with the majority of behaviors measured (Kurdi et al., 2019). However, a majority of the studies examined were underpowered, highlighting that more research is required to further assess implicit and explicit measures as predictors of behavior.

Understanding Implicit Processes
Consistent with research on the IAT, implicit processes have been likened to simple associations between various products of information processing (frequently, memory of attitudes or stereotypes; Greenwald et al., 2009), which can be especially beneficial in understanding areas of illness identification, response, and treatment behaviors (Orbell & Phillips, 2019). For example, implicit positive attitudes about a medication ("Drug X will help me greatly!") at Moment Y may be associated with a subsequent decision to take medication at that moment. Alternatively, implicit processes are described as wholly functioning executive processes that occur outside awareness, seemingly transforming information to meet the demands of the situation; Dijksterhuis and colleagues (Dijksterhuis & Aarts, 2010; Dijksterhuis & Nordgren, 2006) called this incubation or the sleep-on-it effect. A person, for example, may spontaneously seem to understand the costs and benefits of a decision about a health behavior, even though they had been stumped in the past.

Although not well-developed for health decisions, some research has found associations between implicit attitudes and health decisions and behaviors. One main area of focus consists of food choice and consumption (Friese et al., 2008) in which a meta-analysis found that a variety of interventions targeted toward implicit processes were positively associated with effects on eating behavior (Aulbach et al., 2019). Research has suggested similar findings regarding health decisions and adolescents' impulsive school behavior (Navarick, 2004), condom use (Broaddus, 2009; Ellis et al., 2016), and marijuana consumption (Ramirez et al., 2020; Scott-Sheldon, 2006). Physical exercise is an area of research that has demonstrated rapid growth in literature examining implicit attitudes of health behavior; a meta-analysis of 26 studies found implicit attitudes and physical activity to have a small but significant correlation (Chevance et al., 2019). There is also a fairly extensive body of research that has examined implicit reactions related to addictions. Implicit positive reactions to alcohol significantly predicted drinking in adolescents (Thush & Wiers, 2007), and stronger implicit associations of alcohol with positive arousal were related to increased alcohol use (Houben et al., 2009). Negative implicit attitudes toward smoking have been associated with abstinence (Kahler et al., 2007) and positive behavior change (Lee et al., 2018) independent of explicit attitudes, and have predicted lower levels of craving and tobacco dependence (Waters et al., 2007).

Another study examined explicit versus implicit attitudes to psychiatric medication among 85 people with schizophrenia and other psychiatric disabilities (Rüsch et al., 2009). Explicit, but not implicit, positive attitudes to psychiatric medication predicted higher self-reported medication use. However, implicit, not explicit, positive attitudes to medication predicted stronger insight into having a mental illness and stronger perceived need for treatment. Implicit and explicit attitudes were not correlated, though, suggesting that the two represent distinct constructs. That study indicated that implicit attitudes to treatment can be measured and can explain variance of treatment-related variables independent of explicit attitudes. The effect of implicit attitudes on treatment-related cognitions and behaviors needs to continue to be examined in future research.

Implicit processes help explain more nuanced components of Sylvia's behaviors. As a rational patient, Sylvia has an identified goal ("I want to meet with my job coach to pursue employment"); however, she may hold implicit negative attitudes about working (e.g., working is too difficult, it isn't worth the time or energy that is required) or her ability to perform in a job (e.g., "I'm too lazy to have a job," "I don't work as fast as others") based on her experiences in previous employment. Sylvia's beliefs can affect her ability to follow through with her intended behavior of attending the scheduled meeting with her job coach. Therefore, identifying and understanding Sylvia's implicit attitudes regarding employment may be especially informative and beneficial to the health care provider supporting Sylvia in achieving her goals.

Influencing Implicit Processes

Some practice-oriented clinical approaches (POCAs) seem to improve largely automated, everyday health behaviors (Sritharan & Gawronski, 2010). The collaborative process of SDM offers space for the patient and health care provider to create plans in advance and implement these POCAs. In turn, this allows for the ability to improve health decisions far beyond the initial process of the rational patient, who weighs pros and cons of available options.

Promising research has explored intervention-based studies of attentional bias and implicit attitudes through the use of practice-based training (Sheeran et al., 2013). An intervention among older adults to improve blood glucose monitoring successfully used detailed implementation plans, including imagination techniques, to enhance decision making during largely automated daily routines of participants (L. L. Liu & Park, 2004). In a study examining the effect of food labels on food choice and attitudes, findings suggested that repeated exposure to health warning labels may alter the association between implicit attitudes and food choices (Asbridge et al., 2021). Similarly, a study pairing images of health consequences with specific energy-dense snack foods was found to change implicit attitudes such that individuals exposed to this condition were more likely to select fruit as opposed to snack options (Hollands et al., 2011). A smoking cessation trial found an association between implicit smoking attitudes and smoking behavior with negative changes in attitude correlating with positive changes in smoking behavior outcomes (Lee et al., 2018). In a laboratory-based setting, Wiers and colleagues (2010) used an evaluative conditioning procedure— the repeated pairing of alcohol-related and negative stimuli—to modify implicit attitudes related to alcohol abuse. The thought was that pairing alcohol-related stimuli with words or pictures of negative valence would lead to a new affective association with the attitude object. Evaluative conditioning was shown to induce more negative implicit attitudes, less alcohol consumption, and less craving (Houben, Havermans, & Wiers, 2010; Houben, Schoenmakers, & Wiers, 2010). Another study involved approach reactions and avoidance reactions with a computer joystick to alcohol-related stimuli; participants learned avoidance behaviors and unlearned approach behaviors, which, in turn, predicted subsequent alcohol consumption (Wiers et al., 2010). Although implicit reactions may be improved by evaluative conditioning, investigators cautioned that such interventions are only effective when also targeting explicit attitudes; research suggested the benefit of designing interventions that separately target implicit and explicit attitudes (Mattavelli et al., 2017). The same is likely to apply to interventions meant to affect health and rehabilitation decisions in the SDM process.

The preceding approaches, such as using detailed implementation plans, can be applied in Sylvia's case to improve decision making. Sylvia and her health care provider work together to identify implicit attitudes and talk through potential challenges that may arise on the day of and days leading up to meeting with her job coach (e.g., beliefs of inadequacy and unpreparedness). By collaboratively working to create detailed plans and develop a routine for the upcoming week (e.g., preselect the outfit that will be worn on the day of the meeting, go to sleep at 10 p.m., wake up at 7 a.m., leave the house by 12 p.m. on Wednesday), they are able to account for implicit processes that interfere with Sylvia's ability to follow through with meeting with her job coach.

Immediate Processes: Greater Effect on Health Decisions and Behaviors

The idea of rational health decision making sometimes suggests health and treatment are discrete phenomena with clear beginning and end points. This may frame treatment participation as an outcome, which misguides some researchers into a one-time end measurement. However, the process is much more complex, and the use of SDM helps the patient in navigating this complexity. Pescosolido (1992) redefined finite health decision and beliefs as more of a continuous and dynamic experience. Viewing treatment decisions and behaviors as one of many experiences on a health care trajectory frames the experience in terms of the stream of social life and interactions. Assessment of single and relatively distant health decisions fails to capture the phenomenon of actually doing treatment within the context of daily life. Experiences are dynamic and influenced by ever changing social forces. External and internal mediators affect relationships between health decisions, addressing similar needs at different times. The TRA and TPB have specifically focused on the immediacy of decisions and behaviors (Ajzen, 1988; Ajzen & Fishbein, 1980).

Understanding the Immediate Context

Notably, these paradigms do not explain behaviors per se but behavioral intentions. Behavior intentions are most likely to reflect actual behavior when the intention occurs relatively soon before the setting and time in which the behavior was meant to happen. In terms of health behavior, research has shown that recollections of painful/unpleasant medical procedures are strongly influenced by the most recent or end characteristics of the procedure (Redelmeier & Kahneman, 1996; Redelmeier et al., 2003). Ironically, people seem to favor longer procedures if they entail less discomfort at the end step, even if earlier steps produced notable pain intensity (Kahneman et al., 1993; Redelmeier et al., 2003). Additionally, pain recall and future pain reporting is suggested to be influenced by cognitive processes in which remembered pain was reported as higher than an individual's initial level of reported pain (Gedney & Logan, 2006), further highlighting the role of immediate processes (current memory of pain experience) in influencing distant reporting experiences.

The significance of momentary characteristics of a procedure affecting behaviors is typically overlooked in research examining predictors of "poor" decisions: long-term, fixed variables, such as cognitive characteristics, gender, age, socioeconomic status, and type of illness (DiMatteo, 2004; DiMatteo et al., 2002; Gonzalez et al., 2008; Grenard et al., 2011). Although the study of stable variables may be useful for determining systemic resource allocation and preemptive/prevention efforts in populations that undermine health decisions, SDM often requires ongoing daily efforts that are facilitated or hindered by one's immediate context. Health decisions are not isolated decisions with a predetermined aftermath. Rather, decision making is a process that occurs in ever changing intrapersonal, interpersonal, and physical conditions that may affect one's ability or motivation to engage in, or curtail, daily behaviors.

Considering the effect of immediate processes on behavior, a number of factors could be explored in the example of Sylvia. Let's consider an instance in which Sylvia gets into an argument with her husband 15 minutes before she is supposed to leave for her meeting. Having lost track of time because of the argument, Sylvia realizes she is now late for her meeting. Although she had a behavioral intention (leave the house at 12 p.m. to arrive on time for her meeting at 1 p.m.), factors came up immediately preceding the time that she was supposed to leave the house, ultimately preventing her from implementing her intended behavior.

Influencing the Immediate Context

Correlational or retrospective designs are incapable of capturing the dynamic nature of health decisions and behaviors or of identifying the role that immediate and contextual factors may play. Correlational models, for example, provide snapshots of one's health decisions in context but are ill-equipped to examine fluctuating behavior or contextually changing factors. A retrospective view encompasses periods in which dynamic processes likely took place, but that view relies on research participants' ability to recall and summarize their experiences accurately, a process shown to produce biased reports and demonstrate limitations in identifying variability in an individual's experience over time when compared with real-time ratings (Ben-Zeev & Young, 2010; Ben-Zeev et al., 2009, 2012; Ebner-Priemer et al., 2006; Prince et al., 2020).

Experience-sampling methods (ESMs) offer a measurement model that may be effective in capturing the ebb and flow of behaviors and allows for the ability to examine possible effects of immediate contextual factors (Csikszentmihalyi & Larson, 1987), providing additional insight that can be applied to the SDM process. ESM (also known as ambulatory assessment or ecological momentary assessment) is an intensive repeated measures strategy that uses an electronic device to prompt participants to complete self-report questionnaires about their immediate thoughts, feelings, bodily sensations, activities, and settings in real-time multiple times a day. Data collected from ESM reflect an individual's immediate or most recent state within the context and flow of daily experience, facilitating the study of microprocesses that influence behavior in real-world contexts (Beal, 2015; Shiffman et al., 2008). With real-time data capture, researchers can map the temporal sequence or co-occurrence of events over a given period of data collection, identifying immediate or short-term relationships between variables and within individuals (Ebner-Priemer et al., 2009).

A recent meta-analysis highlighted the use of ESM in understanding commonly studied contextual factors (e.g., feeling states, social influences, motivation/goals) of various health-related behaviors (Perski et al., 2022). Specifically, recent studies using this approach have produced some insights into relationships between immediate contextual factors and health-related behaviors, including cigarette smoking in individuals attempting to quit (Perski et al., 2023; Shiffman & Kirchner, 2009), physical activity in adolescents (Bourke et al., 2022) and older adults (Dunton et al., 2009; Hevel et al., 2021), self-injurious behaviors (Brown et al., 2022; Nock et al., 2009; Rodríguez-Blanco et al., 2018), and self-medication of symptoms via substance use in schizophrenia (Swendsen et al., 2011).

Research has also explored the utility of mobile technologies for ecological momentary interventions (EMIs) that provide real-time, real-world support for a variety of health decisions (Depp et al., 2010; Heron & Smyth, 2010). For example, providers give patients personal digital assistants (PDAs) that provide repeated, real-time reminders of previously agreed on health decisions. Time, place, and content of reminders are set as an algorithm based on previous ESM findings. These can be further enhanced with interactive voice response systems integrated into EMI strategies to improve the quality and diversity of cues (Freedman et al., 2006; Levin & Levin, 2006). Advancements in technology have contributed to a growing body of methods for collecting real-time data and implementing interventions by use of passive (e.g., sensors, phone, app data) or active (e.g., diary techniques) methods (Schick et al., 2023). Evidence suggests EMIs may be beneficial in targeting smoking cessation (Eghdami et al., 2023), substance use disorder (Carreiro et al., 2020), and a broad range of mental health disorders (Balaskas et al., 2021) and may prove feasible, acceptable, and efficacious for enhancing health decisions and behaviors across a variety of clinical populations. EMIs can be used to target a range of mental health disorders and provide easily accessible mental health support through implementation of evidence-based methods that are well received by the individuals using them (Marciniak et al., 2020).

Using EMIs can help support Sylvia's adherence to her decision. Offering EMI tools (e.g., PDA) during Sylvia's SDM meeting provides her with the assistance needed to follow through with attending her meeting, even when more immediate factors arise. Having set cues and reminders (e.g., leave the house at 12 p.m.) helps minimize the effect of immediate factors that disrupt her intended behavior, ultimately increasing adherence.

Emotions Influencing Many Health Decisions

Emotions influence health decision making independent of cognition both directly and indirectly, which seemingly challenges a rational patient. First, emotions have been likened to motivation, with people making specific health decisions to obtain or avoid consequences of emotions that accompany those decisions. In this way, motivation activates the decision-making task. Second, research has found the interoceptive sequelae of emotions may have direct, not cognitively mediated, effects on processes, such as SDM. In part, this is an arousal function, a more nonspecific version of psychological activation.

Emotions Motivating Health Decisions

Daniel Kahneman (1999) proposed hedonic theory to argue that perceived utility of a decision or behavior is influenced by the emotional response to the experience, which subsequently affects whether said decision or behavior will be repeated. Consistent with this theory, a majority of the research has examined and demonstrated that affect and emotions correspond with a range of health decisions with some (negatively valenced) seeming to undermine health decisions, whereas others (more positively charged) enhance decisions (Magai et al., 2007; Williams & Evans, 2014). Affect can be viewed as influencing health via direct or indirect pathways (DeSteno et al., 2013). Direct effects consider the impact of current affective states on physiological changes and responses (e.g., stress affecting cardiac functioning and blood pressure, directly affecting health outcomes), whereas indirect effects concern the influence of affect on health decisions and behaviors (e.g., affect influencing risk perception and contributing towards an individual's decision in seeking treatment or screenings, indirectly contributing to health outcomes; Magnan et al., 2017). Hedonic theory has been used to understand the effects of emotion on health conditions and behavior, including obesity (Cota et al., 2006; Mela, 2006; Stroebe, 2022), smoking (Blendy et al., 2005; Dawkins et al., 2007; Shiffman & Terhorst, 2017), substance abuse (Berridge, 2007; Stevens et al., 2007), and exercise (Box & Petruzzello, 2020; Murphy & Eaves, 2016; Williams, 2008). Therefore, hedonic theory informs SDM in understanding that emotions contribute to the initiation and progress of the decision-making process, suggesting the rational process of making decisions is not the sole contributor.

Research has fairly consistently shown that depression undermines treatment decisions; one meta-analysis yielded an odds ratio greater than 3 (DiMatteo et al., 2000), and another yielded an odds ratio of 1.76 for medication adherence in individuals with chronic disease (Grenard et al., 2011). People who are depressed are less likely to adhere to hypertensive (Kariis et al., 2023; Q. Liu et al., 2022), asthma (Dong et al., 2024) and human immunodeficiency virus (HIV; Ogburn et al., 2019; Tao et al., 2018) medication prescriptions as well as renal dialysis (Brownbridge & Fielding, 1994; Nabolsi et al., 2015; Oh et al., 2013), mammography or other procedures for breast cancer (Magai et al., 2007; Park et al., 2020), and medication treatments for diabetes (Escobar Florez et al., 2021; Kalsekar et al., 2006) and cancer (Irwin & Johnson, 2015).

Research on the effects of anxiety, which would seem to be similarly valenced, is mixed showing the complexity of linking decision making to quality of negative affect. Psychological distress has been found to be associated with certain factors (e.g., medication adherence) in kidney transplant patients (Pabst et al., 2015) but not others (e.g., lifestyle adherence) in patients with heart failure (Eisele et al., 2020). Consider health decisions about interventions related to breast cancer (Magai et al., 2007). A recent systematic review highlighted fear, anxiety, worry, and embarrassment as main perceived barriers to breast cancer screenings with fear also serving as a motivational factor in screening (Tavakoli et al., 2024). There is a significant relationship between cancer fear and screening but, interestingly, a significant and inverse relationship between fear related to hospitalization, surgery, or mammography screening (Consedine et al., 2004). People who are highly emotional and concerned about pain are less likely to adhere to pharmacological treatment for chronic pain (Nicklas et al., 2010). A particularly social aspect of anxiety—embarrassment—is also related to health decisions. People will avoid illness screening or other aspects of treatment to escape feelings of fear and worry in relation to the stigma of that illness (Corrigan, 2004; Garbers et al., 2003; Li et al., 2022; O'Malley et al., 2023). Being able to identify and anticipate avoidance of behaviors based on emotional experiences is helpful to the health care provider assisting the patient in not only making a decision but also completing the behaviors necessary to adhere to their decision. Discussing emotions as they relate to patient-identified goals can be a useful indicator of behavioral outcomes.

Interoception and Arousal

Interoception is defined as sensitivity to stimuli originating within the body, which includes a variety of systems (e.g., cardiovascular, endocrine, gastrointestinal, respiratory, urogenital) that contribute to emotional feelings (Nayok et al., 2023). It has also broadly been equated to visceral or somatic markers and associated with constructs related to physiological arousal and activation. Significant research has examined the relationship between proxies of interoception and emotional arousal. Studies have shown that better interoceptive accuracy (e.g., heartbeat detection) translates into greater intensity of affect perception (Coll et al., 2021; Parrinello et al., 2022). More relevant to the point here, research examining the relationship among interoception, arousal, and decision making has shown visceral effects of emotion partially influence decision making via its effect on perceived reinforcement and punishment of outcomes of that decision (Damasio, 1994; Dunn et al., 2010; Naqvi & Bechara, 2009). Specifically, greater anticipatory skin conductance responses have been associated with disadvantageous decision making compared with advantageous decision-making choices (Guillaume et al., 2009). These kinds of processes specifically influence health-related decision making (E. E. Hall et al., 2010; Jollant et al., 2010). Indeed, research has identified a slew of psychological processes (e.g., affective predictions, current emotional states, information perceived and integrated from the body, reflection and integration of appraisals) relevant to health decision making that are emotionally driven outside of awareness (Cunningham et al., 2013). Specific examples of information processing identified within research consists of threat appraisal (Adolphs et al., 2005; Wood & Della-Monica, 2015), others' traits (Azevedo et al., 2023; Willis & Todorov, 2006; Winston et al., 2002), and social rewards (Cloutier et al., 2008; Liang et al., 2010).

In what ways are Sylvia's emotions and interoceptive awareness affecting her decision making? When Sylvia makes the decision to schedule a meeting with her job coach, fear could serve as a strong motivation in arriving at her decision because she could be worried about negative outcomes (e.g., financial concerns) if she does not find a job. Additional concerns of embarrassment may arise when she physically attends the meeting with her job coach resulting from fear that she will be judged for getting fired from her previous job and worrying about how she will be able to perform in her next job. Interoceptive experiences, such as increased heart rate and skin conductance, correspond with Sylvia's emotions of fear and embarrassment, heightening her perception of emotions and ultimately affecting her decisions and potential avoidance behaviors.

One of the goals of many cognitive therapies is to teach people how to manage emotions by reframing the appraisals that correspond with them. In this light, cognitive therapy may help the rational patient. Alternatively, knowledge that emotions are independent psychological processes that often affect human behavior and are experienced separate from cognition has significantly influenced relatively recent and innovative perspectives about change strategies. Two principles have emerged to expand the potential of cognitive behavior therapy (CBT): (a) acceptance and (b) mindfulness, which have been identified in treatment interventions of acceptance and commitment therapy and dialectical behavior therapy.

Acceptance suggests hurtful psychiatric problems and symptoms can be overcome, not by fighting symptoms per se, but by recognizing those symptoms and accepting them as an authentic part of the person's condition at that moment (Hayes et al., 1999). Hence, contrary to many CBT approaches suggesting that negative emotional reactions to health should somehow be controlled, notions of acceptance encourage the person to recognize the positive or negatively valenced affect in response to the health condition or treatment and to use these emotional reactions to better understand and experience the event. Mindfulness through meditation is a tool that promotes acceptance and health decision making (Goldberg et al., 2023; Kabat-Zinn, 2001; Linehan, 1993). Mindfulness is an attempt to experience psychological phenomena unfettered by behavior or cognitions. It is the self-regulation and orientation of attention focused on the present moment with curiosity and openness (Bishop et al., 2004).

Only recently has research proposed or examined how therapies incorporating acceptance and mindfulness affect health decisions. Exploring how these strategies can be applied within the SDM process can be beneficial in enhancing patients' decisions and behaviors. A number of research articles have identified acceptance and commitment therapy–based interventions and protocols designed to target medication adherence in women with breast cancer who are undergoing adjuvant endocrine therapy; however, these studies focused on identifying protocols for pilot trials and did not produce results regarding the implementation of the interventions themselves (Green et al., 2022; L. H. Hall et al., 2022; Smith et al., 2022, 2023). In individuals with HIV, acceptance and disclosure of HIV status may be helpful in managing treatment retention; one pilot randomized clinical trial study identified that HIV patients assigned to an acceptance-based behavior therapy group had a higher likelihood of care retention compared with a group receiving treatment as usual (Moitra et al., 2017).

Mindfulness may be an important intervention target in enhancing health decision making. One study identified higher smoking frequency in those with low trait compared with high trait–level mindfulness, suggesting mindfulness treatment targets may help protect against risk decision-making processes (Black et al., 2012). Mindfulness interventions may be a helpful tool in addressing health related decision making when certain factors are involved. Findings have indicated that individuals presented with colorectal cancer screening and treatment scenarios who scored higher on measures of nonjudging mindfulness demonstrated less disgust compared with individuals with lower mindfulness (Reynolds et al., 2014). Additionally, results were suggestive that when making decisions, those with higher mindfulness may use experiences of disgust to help inform decisions, whereas those with lower mindfulness may ignore emotional experiences. Although more research is certainly needed regarding the integration of mindfulness and acceptance in treatment, these are promising areas of focus in enhancing health-related decisions and behaviors.

In the case of Sylvia, having a health care provider work with her in the SDM process to implement mindfulness strategies can help her become more aware of her emotions, identify interoceptive cues, and better manage reactions that are affecting her decision making.

CONCLUSION

SDM is an important example of a broader collection of health-related decisions and behaviors. The rational patient is one popular paradigm for understanding health decisions and behaviors, including largely cognitive behavioral methods to affect the deliberative decision maker. However, we have identified several limitations to that approach.

We do not mean to dismiss rational actor models; social psychologists have not done so. One solution has been dual-process paradigms that have sought to describe the interaction of explicit and implicit processes in everyday behavior (Chaiken & Trope, 1999). The MODE (motivation and opportunity as determinants) model has been proposed as an example of such integration (Fazio, 1990; Fazio & Towles-Schwen, 1999; Olson & Fazio, 2008). Given the effort that reflection requires in explicit processes, some motivation is required to be deliberative in behaviors. When there are no perceived costs or benefits to a health behavior like taking medications, for example, there is no motivation to be deliberative or effortful in considerations. Deliberating cost alone is insufficient for explicit processes (Fazio, 1990; Fazio & Towles-Schwen, 1999; Olson & Fazio, 2008). Time and resources to deliberate—what the MODE model calls opportunity—must also be available. Situations requiring a rapid response fail to provide the time the person needs to carefully consider multiple contingencies and take action. Hence, the person confronted by unexpected side effects of a medication moments before having to dash out of the apartment for work is more likely to rely on implicit processes. Although social psychologists continue to develop more advanced dual process models as research matures, the morale remains the same: It is the integration of the rational patient paradigm and the addenda outlined in this chapter that provide the most complete picture of health decisions and behaviors.

The rational patient model suggests that health decisions are made deliberatively through careful consideration of advantages and disadvantages; however, we highlighted that significant cognitive processes occur implicitly and potentially outside awareness. These might be simple associations between two constructs—taking medication is bad—or may represent totally separate executive processes outside awareness—Dijksterhuis and Aarts's (2010) sleep-on-it effect. Theories and measurement models related to the IAT and corresponding POCAs continue to describe and expand on the effect of the implicit relationship between health decisions and satisfaction. We also identified that the person is both planful as well as influenced by the immediate exigencies, factors that often differ from the consideration of days earlier. Health behavior requires ongoing daily effort to realize and carry out a health plan. Research relying on ESMs and EMIs has helped to understand the immediacy of influences and ways to affect them.

In this chapter, we also considered that the rational patient is not always a cool operator who acts on decisions divorced from emotion. Instead, research shows that decision making is oftentimes a hot process with emotions occurring both explicitly (as inhibitors of motivators for specific decisions) and implicitly (interoceptive and arousing processes that may orient the person to different decisions and behaviors). The evolution of clinical therapies to include mindfulness and acceptance have begun to demonstrate potential utility in improving satisfaction with health decisions.

REFERENCES

Adolphs, R., Gosselin, F., Buchanan, T. W., Tranel, D., Schyns, P., & Damasio, A. R. (2005). A mechanism for impaired fear recognition after amygdala damage. *Nature, 433*(7021), 68–72. https://doi.org/10.1038/nature03086

Ajzen, I. (1988). *Attitudes, personality, and behavior.* Open University Press.

Ajzen, I., & Fishbein, M. (1980). *Understanding attitudes and predicting social behavior.* Prentice-Hall.

Armitage, C. J., & Conner, M. (2000). Attitudinal ambivalence: A test of three key hypotheses. *Personality and Social Psychology Bulletin, 26*(11), 1421–1432. https://doi.org/10.1177/0146167200263009

Asbridge, S. C. M., Pechey, E., Marteau, T. M., & Hollands, G. J. (2021). Effects of pairing health warning labels with energy-dense snack foods on food choice and attitudes: Online experimental study. *Appetite, 160,* Article 105090. https://doi.org/10.1016/j.appet.2020.105090

Aulbach, M. B., Knittle, K., & Haukkala, A. (2019). Implicit process interventions in eating behaviour: A meta-analysis examining mediators and moderators. *Health Psychology Review, 13*(2), 179–208. https://doi.org/10.1080/17437199.2019.1571933

Azevedo, R. T., von Mohr, M., & Tsakiris, M. (2023). From the viscera to first impressions: Phase-dependent cardio-visual signals bias the perceived trustworthiness of faces. *Psychological Science, 34*(1), 120–131. https://doi.org/10.1177/09567976221131519

Balaskas, A., Schueller, S. M., Cox, A. L., & Doherty, G. (2021). Ecological momentary interventions for mental health: A scoping review. *PLOS ONE, 16*(3), e0248152. https://doi.org/10.1371/journal.pone.0248152

Bandura, A. (1977). *Social learning theory.* General Learning Press.

Bandura, A. (1986). *Social foundations of thought and action: A social cognitive theory.* Prentice-Hall.

Bargh, J. A. (1994). The four horsemen of automaticity: Awareness, intention, efficiency, and control in social cognition. In R. S. Wyer & T. K. Srull (Eds.), *Handbook of social cognition* (Vol. 2, pp. 1–40). Lawrence Erlbaum Associates.

Beal, D. J. (2015). ESM 2.0: State of the art and future potential of experience sampling methods in organizational research. *Annual Review of Organizational Psychology and Organizational Behavior, 2*(1), 383–407. https://doi.org/10.1146/annurev-orgpsych-032414-111335

Ben-Zeev, D., McHugo, G. J., Xie, H., Dobbins, K., & Young, M. A. (2012). Comparing retrospective reports to real-time/real-place mobile assessments in individuals with schizophrenia and a nonclinical comparison group. *Schizophrenia Bulletin, 38*(3), 396–404. https://doi.org/10.1093/schbul/sbr171

Ben-Zeev, D., & Young, M. A. (2010). Accuracy of hospitalized depressed patients' and healthy controls' retrospective symptom reports: An experience sampling study. *Journal of Nervous and Mental Disease, 198*(4), 280–285. https://doi.org/10.1097/NMD.0b013e3181d6141f

Ben-Zeev, D., Young, M. A., & Madsen, J. W. (2009). Retrospective recall of affect in clinically depressed individuals and controls. *Cognition and Emotion, 23*(5), 1021–1040. https://doi.org/10.1080/02699930802607937

Berridge, K. C. (2007). The debate over dopamine's role in reward: The case for incentive salience. *Psychopharmacology, 191*(3), 391–431. https://doi.org/10.1007/s00213-006-0578-x

Bickel, W. K., Moody, L., & Higgins, S. T. (2016). Some current dimensions of the behavioral economics of health-related behavior change. *Preventive Medicine, 92*, 16–23. https://doi.org/10.1016/j.ypmed.2016.06.002

Bickel, W. K., & Vuchinich, R. E. (Eds.). (2000). *Reframing health behavior change with behavioral economics.* Lawrence Erlbaum Associates Publishers. https://doi.org/10.4324/9781410605061

Bishop, S. R., Lau, M., Shapiro, S., Carlson, L., Anderson, N. D., Carmody, J., Segal, Z. V., Abbey, S., Speca, M., Velting, D., & Devins, G. (2004). Mindfulness: A proposed operational definition. *Clinical Psychology, 11*(3), 230–241. https://doi.org/10.1093/clipsy.bph077

Black, D. S., Sussman, S., Johnson, C. A., & Milam, J. (2012). Trait mindfulness helps shield decision-making from translating into health-risk behavior. *The Journal of Adolescent Health, 51*(6), 588–592. https://doi.org/10.1016/j.jadohealth.2012.03.011

Blendy, J. A., Strasser, A., Walters, C. L., Perkins, K. A., Patterson, F., Berkowitz, R., & Lerman, C. (2005). Reduced nicotine reward in obesity: Cross-comparison in human and mouse. *Psychopharmacology, 180*(2), 306–315. https://doi.org/10.1007/s00213-005-2167-9

Bourke, M., Patten, R. K., Hilland, T. A., & Craike, M. (2022). Within-person associations between physical and social contexts with movement behavior compositions in adolescents: An ecological momentary assessment study using a compositional data analysis approach. *Journal of Physical Activity & Health, 19*(9), 615–622. https://doi.org/10.1123/jpah.2022-0233

Box, A. G., & Petruzzello, S. J. (2020). Why do they do it? Differences in high-intensity exercise-affect between those with higher and lower intensity preference and tolerance. *Psychology of Sport and Exercise, 47*, Article 101521. https://doi.org/10.1016/j.psychsport.2019.04.011

Broaddus, M. (2009). *Multidimensional implicit and explicit condom attitudes: Structure and implications for health messages* (Publication No. 3315812) [Doctoral dissertation, University of Colorado]. ProQuest Dissertations and Theses Global.

Brown, A. C., Dhingra, K., Brown, T. D., Danquah, A. N., & Taylor, P. J. (2022). A systematic review of the relationship between momentary emotional states and nonsuicidal self-injurious thoughts and behaviours. *Psychology and Psychotherapy: Theory, Research and Practice, 95*(3), 754–780. https://doi.org/10.1111/papt.12397

Brownbridge, G., & Fielding, D. M. (1994). Psychosocial adjustment and adherence to dialysis treatment regimes. *Pediatric Nephrology, 8*(6), 744–749. https://doi.org/10.1007/BF00869109

Carpenter, C. J. (2010). A meta-analysis of the effectiveness of health belief model variables in predicting behavior. *Health Communication, 25*(8), 661–669. https://doi.org/10.1080/10410236.2010.521906

Carreiro, S., Newcomb, M., Leach, R., Ostrowski, S., Boudreaux, E. D., & Amante, D. (2020). Current reporting of usability and impact of mHealth interventions for substance use disorder: A systematic review. *Drug and Alcohol Dependence, 215,* Article 108201. https://doi.org/10.1016/j.drugalcdep.2020.108201

Chaiken, S., & Trope, Y. (1999). *Dual-process theories in social psychology.* The Guilford Press.

Champion, V. L., & Skinner, C. S. (2008). The health belief model. In K. Glanz, B. K. Rimer, & K. Viswanath (Eds.), *Health behavior and health education: Theory, research, and practice* (4th ed., pp. 45–65). Jossey-Bass/Wiley.

Chevance, G., Bernard, P., Chamberland, P. E., & Rebar, A. (2019). The association between implicit attitudes toward physical activity and physical activity behaviour: A systematic review and correlational meta-analysis. *Health Psychology Review, 13*(3), 248–276. https://doi.org/10.1080/17437199.2019.1618726

Cloutier, J., Heatherton, T. F., Whalen, P. J., & Kelley, W. M. (2008). Are attractive people rewarding? Sex differences in the neural substrates of facial attractiveness. *Journal of Cognitive Neuroscience, 20*(6), 941–951. https://doi.org/10.1162/jocn.2008.20062

Coll, M. P., Hobson, H., Bird, G., & Murphy, J. (2021). Systematic review and meta-analysis of the relationship between the heartbeat-evoked potential and interoception. *Neuroscience and Biobehavioral Reviews, 122,* 190–200. https://doi.org/10.1016/j.neubiorev.2020.12.012

Conner, M., & Norman, P. (Eds.). (2005). *Predicting health behaviour: A social cognition approach* (2nd ed.). Open University Press.

Consedine, N. S., Magai, C., Krivoshekova, Y. S., Ryzewicz, L., & Neugut, A. I. (2004). Fear, anxiety, worry, and breast cancer screening behavior: A critical review. *Cancer Epidemiology, Biomarkers & Prevention, 13*(4), 501–510. https://doi.org/10.1158/1055-9965.501.13.4

Corrigan, P. (2004). How stigma interferes with mental health care. *American Psychologist, 59*(7), 614–625. https://doi.org/10.1037/0003-066X.59.7.614

Cota, D., Tschöp, M. H., Horvath, T. L., & Levine, A. S. (2006). Cannabinoids, opioids and eating behavior: The molecular face of hedonism? *Brain Research Reviews, 51*(1), 85–107. https://doi.org/10.1016/j.brainresrev.2005.10.004

Csikszentmihalyi, M., & Larson, R. (1987). Validity and reliability of the experience-sampling method. *Journal of Nervous and Mental Disease, 175*(9), 526–536. https://doi.org/10.1097/00005053-198709000-00004

Cunningham, W. A., Dunfield, K. A., & Stillman, P. E. (2013). Emotional states from affective dynamics. *Emotion Review, 5*(4), 344–355. https://doi.org/10.1177/1754073913489749

Damasio, A. R. (1994). *Descartes' error: Emotion, reason, and the human brain.* Grosset/Putnam.

Dawkins, L., Acaster, S., & Powell, J. H. (2007). The effects of smoking and abstinence on experience of happiness and sadness in response to positively valenced, negatively valenced, and neutral film clips. *Addictive Behaviors, 32*(2), 425–431. https://doi.org/10.1016/j.addbeh.2006.05.010

Depp, C. A., Mausbach, B., Granholm, E., Cardenas, V., Ben-Zeev, D., Patterson, T. L., Lebowitz, B. D., & Jeste, D. V. (2010). Mobile interventions for severe mental illness: Design and preliminary data from three approaches. *Journal of Nervous and Mental Disease, 198*(10), 715–721. https://doi.org/10.1097/NMD.0b013e3181f49ea3

DeSteno, D., Gross, J. J., & Kubzansky, L. (2013). Affective science and health: The importance of emotion and emotion regulation. *Health Psychology, 32*(5), 474–486. https://doi.org/10.1037/a0030259

Dijksterhuis, A., & Aarts, H. (2010). Goals, attention, and (un)consciousness. *Annual Review of Psychology, 61*(1), 467–490. https://doi.org/10.1146/annurev.psych. 093008.100445

Dijksterhuis, A., & Nordgren, L. F. (2006). A theory of unconscious thought. *Perspectives on Psychological Science, 1*(2), 95–109. https://doi.org/10.1111/j.1745-6916. 2006.00007.x

DiMatteo, M. R. (2004). Social support and patient adherence to medical treatment: A meta-analysis. *Health Psychology, 23*(2), 207–218. https://doi.org/10.1037/ 0278-6133.23.2.207

DiMatteo, M. R., Giordani, P. J., Lepper, H. S., & Croghan, T. W. (2002). Patient adherence and medical treatment outcomes: A meta-analysis. *Medical Care, 40*(9), 794–811. https://doi.org/10.1097/00005650-200209000-00009

DiMatteo, M. R., Lepper, H. S., & Croghan, T. W. (2000). Depression is a risk factor for noncompliance with medical treatment: Meta-analysis of the effects of anxiety and depression on patient adherence. *Archives of Internal Medicine, 160*(14), 2101–2107. https://doi.org/10.1001/archinte.160.14.2101

Dong, R., Sun, S., Sun, Y., Wang, Y., & Zhang, X. (2024). The association of depressive symptoms and medication adherence in asthma patients: The mediation effect of medication beliefs. *Research in Social and Administrative Pharmacy, 20*(3), 335–344. https://doi.org/10.1016/j.sapharm.2023.12.002

Dunn, B. D., Galton, H. C., Morgan, R., Evans, D., Oliver, C., Meyer, M., Cusack, R., Lawrence, A. D., & Dalgleish, T. (2010). Listening to your heart: How interoception shapes emotion experience and intuitive decision making. *Psychological Science, 21*(12), 1835–1844. https://doi.org/10.1177/0956797610389191

Dunton, G. F., Atienza, A. A., Castro, C. M., & King, A. C. (2009). Using ecological momentary assessment to examine antecedents and correlates of physical activity bouts in adults age 50+ years: A pilot study. *Annals of Behavioral Medicine, 38*(3), 249–255. https://doi.org/10.1007/s12160-009-9141-4

Dymond, S., May, R. J., Munnelly, A., & Hoon, A. E. (2010). Evaluating the evidence base for relational frame theory: A citation analysis. *The Behavior Analyst, 33*(1), 97–117. https://doi.org/10.1007/BF03392206

Ebner-Priemer, U. W., Eid, M., Kleindienst, N., Stabenow, S., & Trull, T. J. (2009). Analytic strategies for understanding affective (in)stability and other dynamic processes in psychopathology. *Journal of Abnormal Psychology, 118*(1), 195–202. https://doi.org/10.1037/a0014868

Ebner-Priemer, U. W., Kuo, J., Welch, S. S., Thielgen, T., Witte, S., Bohus, M., & Linehan, M. M. (2006). A valence-dependent group-specific recall bias of retrospective self-reports: A study of borderline personality disorder in everyday life. *Journal of Nervous and Mental Disease, 194*(10), 774–779. https://doi.org/10.1097/ 01.nmd.0000239900.46595.72

Eghdami, S., Ahmadkhaniha, H. R., Baradaran, H. R., & Hirbod-Mobarakeh, A. (2023). Ecological momentary interventions for smoking cessation: A systematic review and meta-analysis. *Social Psychiatry and Psychiatric Epidemiology, 58*(10), 1431–1445. https://doi.org/10.1007/s00127-023-02503-2

Eisele, M., Harder, M., Rakebrandt, A., Boczor, S., Marx, G., Blozik, E., Träder, J.-M., Störk, S., Herrmann-Lingen, C., & Scherer, M. (2020). Association of depression and anxiety with adherence in primary care patients with heart failure-cross-sectional results of the observational RECODE-HF cohort study. *Family Practice, 37*(5), 695–702. https://doi.org/10.1093/fampra/cmaa042

Ellis, E. M., Collins, R. L., Homish, G. G., Parks, K. A., & Kiviniemi, M. T. (2016). Perceived controllability of condom use shifts reliance on implicit versus explicit affect. *Health Psychology, 35*(8), 842–846. https://doi.org/10.1037/hea0000336

Escobar Florez, O. E., Aquilera, G., De la Roca-Chiapas, J. M., Macías Cervantes, M. H., & Garay-Sevilla, M. E. (2021). The relationship between psychosocial factors and adherence to treatment in men, premenopausal and menopausal women with Type 2 diabetes mellitus. *Psychology Research and Behavior Management, 14*, 1993–2000. https://doi.org/10.2147/PRBM.S342155

Fazio, R. H. (1990). Multiple processes by which attitudes guide behavior: The MODE model as an integrative framework. In M. P. Zanna (Ed.), *Advances in experimental social psychology* (Vol. 23, pp. 75–109). Academic Press. https://doi.org/10.1016/S0065-2601(08)60318-4

Fazio, R. H., & Towles-Schwen, T. (1999). The MODE model of attitude-behavior processes. In S. Chaiken & Y. Trope (Eds.), *Dual-process theories in social psychology* (pp. 97–116). The Guilford Press.

Fishbein, M., & Ajzen, I. (1975). *Belief, attitude, intention, and behavior.* Addison-Wesley.

Floyd, D. L., Prentice-Dunn, S., & Rogers, R. W. (2000). A meta-analysis of research on protection motivation theory. *Journal of Applied Social Psychology, 30*(2), 407–429. https://doi.org/10.1111/j.1559-1816.2000.tb02323.x

Freedman, M. J., Lester, K. M., McNamara, C., Milby, J. B., & Schumacher, J. E. (2006). Cell phones for ecological momentary assessment with cocaine-addicted homeless patients in treatment. *Journal of Substance Abuse Treatment, 30*(2), 105–111. https://doi.org/10.1016/j.jsat.2005.10.005

Friedman, D., & Hechter, M. (1988). The contribution of rational choice theory to macrosociological research. *Sociological Theory, 6*(2), 201–218. https://doi.org/10.2307/202116

Friese, M., Hofmann, W., & Wänke, M. (2008). When impulses take over: Moderated predictive validity of explicit and implicit attitude measures in predicting food choice and consumption behaviour. *British Journal of Social Psychology, 47*(3), 397–419. https://doi.org/10.1348/014466607X241540

Garbers, S., Jessop, D. J., Foti, H., Uribelarrea, M., & Chiasson, M. A. (2003). Barriers to breast cancer screening for low-income Mexican and Dominican women in New York City. *Journal of Urban Health, 80*(1), 81–91. https://doi.org/10.1007/PL00022327

Gawronski, B., & Bodenhausen, G. V. (2006). Associative and propositional processes in evaluation: An integrative review of implicit and explicit attitude change. *Psychological Bulletin, 132*(5), 692–731. https://doi.org/10.1037/0033-2909.132.5.692

Gedney, J. J., & Logan, H. (2006). Pain related recall predicts future pain report. *Pain, 121*(1), 69–76. https://doi.org/10.1016/j.pain.2005.12.005

Glanz, K., Rimer, B. K., & Viswanath, K. (Eds.). (2008). *Health behavior and health education: Theory, research, and practice* (4th ed.). Jossey-Bass/Wiley.

Goldberg, S. B., Anders, C., Stuart-Maver, S. L., & Kivlighan, D. M., III. (2023). Meditation, mindfulness, and acceptance methods in psychotherapy: A systematic review. *Psychotherapy Research, 33*(7), 873–885. https://doi.org/10.1080/10503307.2023.2209694

Gonzalez, J. S., Peyrot, M., McCarl, L. A., Collins, E. M., Serpa, L., Mimiaga, M. J., & Safren, S. A. (2008). Depression and diabetes treatment nonadherence: A meta-analysis. *Diabetes Care, 31*(12), 2398–2403. https://doi.org/10.2337/dc08-1341

Green, S. M. C., French, D. P., Graham, C. D., Hall, L. H., Rousseau, N., Foy, R., Clark, J., Parbutt, C., Raine, E., Gardner, B., Velikova, G., Moore, S. J. L., Buxton, J., ROSETA investigators, & Smith, S. G. (2022). Supporting adjuvant endocrine therapy adherence in women with breast cancer: The development of a complex behavioural intervention using intervention mapping guided by the multiphase optimisation strategy. *BMC Health Services Research, 22*(1), 1081. https://doi.org/10.1186/s12913-022-08243-4

Greenwald, A. G., McGhee, D. E., & Schwartz, J. L. K. (1998). Measuring individual differences in implicit cognition: The implicit association test. *Journal of Personality and Social Psychology, 74*(6), 1464–1480. https://doi.org/10.1037/0022-3514.74.6.1464

Greenwald, A. G., & Nosek, B. A. (2009). Attitudinal dissociation: What does it mean? In R. E. Petty, R. H. Fazio, & P. Brinol (Eds.), *Attitudes: Insights from the new implicit measures* (pp. 65–82). Psychology Press.

Greenwald, A. G., Poehlman, T. A., Uhlmann, E. L., & Banaji, M. R. (2009). Understanding and using the Implicit Association Test: III. Meta-analysis of predictive validity. *Journal of Personality and Social Psychology, 97*(1), 17–41. https://doi.org/10.1037/a0015575

Grenard, J. L., Munjas, B. A., Adams, J. L., Suttorp, M., Maglione, M., McGlynn, E. A., & Gellad, W. F. (2011). Depression and medication adherence in the treatment of chronic diseases in the United States: A meta-analysis. *Journal of General Internal Medicine, 26*(10), 1175–1182. https://doi.org/10.1007/s11606-011-1704-y

Guillaume, S., Jollant, F., Jaussent, I., Lawrence, N., Malafosse, A., & Courtet, P. (2009). Somatic markers and explicit knowledge are both involved in decision-making. *Neuropsychologia, 47*(10), 2120–2124. https://doi.org/10.1016/j.neuropsychologia.2009.04.003

Hall, E. E., Ekkekakis, P., & Petruzzello, S. J. (2010). Predicting affective responses to exercise using resting EEG frontal asymmetry: Does intensity matter? *Biological Psychology, 83*(3), 201–206. https://doi.org/10.1016/j.biopsycho.2010.01.001

Hall, L. H., Clark, J., Smith, S. G., Graham, C. D., & the ACTION investigators. (2022). Patient and health care professional co-development of an acceptance and commitment therapy intervention to support hormone therapy decision-making and well-being in women with breast cancer. *Journal of Psychosocial Oncology, 40*(4), 407–424. https://doi.org/10.1080/07347332.2021.1955318

Harrison, J. A., Mullen, P. D., & Green, L. W. (1992). A meta-analysis of studies of the health belief model with adults. *Health Education Research, 7*(1), 107–116. https://doi.org/10.1093/her/7.1.107

Hayes, S. C., Barnes-Holmes, D., & Roche, B. (Eds.). (2001). *Relational frame theory: A post-Skinnerian account of human language and cognition.* Kluwer Academic/Plenum Publishers. https://doi.org/10.1007/b108413

Hayes, S. C., Strosahl, K., & Wilson, K. G. (1999). *Acceptance and commitment therapy: An experiential approach to behavior change.* The Guilford Press.

Heron, K. E., & Smyth, J. M. (2010). Ecological momentary interventions: Incorporating mobile technology into psychosocial and health behaviour treatments. *British Journal of Health Psychology, 15*(1), 1–39. https://doi.org/10.1348/135910709X466063

Hevel, D. J., Drollette, E. S., Dunton, G. F., & Maher, J. P. (2021). Social and physical context moderates older adults' affective responses to sedentary behavior: An ecological momentary assessment study. *The Journals of Gerontology: Series B, 76*(10), 1983–1992. https://doi.org/10.1093/geronb/gbab036

Hollands, G. J., Prestwich, A., & Marteau, T. M. (2011). Using aversive images to enhance healthy food choices and implicit attitudes: An experimental test of evaluative conditioning. *Health Psychology, 30*(2), 195–203. https://doi.org/10.1037/a0022261

Houben, K., Havermans, R. C., & Wiers, R. W. (2010). Learning to dislike alcohol: Conditioning negative implicit attitudes toward alcohol and its effect on drinking behavior. *Psychopharmacology, 211*(1), 79–86. https://doi.org/10.1007/s00213-010-1872-1

Houben, K., Rothermund, K., & Wiers, R. W. (2009). Predicting alcohol use with a recoding-free variant of the Implicit Association Test. *Addictive Behaviors, 34*(5), 487–489. https://doi.org/10.1016/j.addbeh.2008.12.012

Houben, K., Schoenmakers, T. M., & Wiers, R. W. (2010). I didn't feel like drinking but I don't know why: The effects of evaluative conditioning on alcohol-related attitudes, craving and behavior. *Addictive Behaviors, 35*(12), 1161–1163. https://doi.org/10.1016/j.addbeh.2010.08.012

Irwin, M., & Johnson, L. A. (2015). Factors influencing oral adherence: Qualitative metasummary and triangulation with quantitative evidence. *Clinical Journal of Oncology Nursing, 19*(3), 6–30. https://doi.org/10.1188/15.S1.CJON.6-30

Jollant, F., Lawrence, N. S., Olie, E., O'Daly, O., Malafosse, A., Courtet, P., & Phillips, M. L. (2010). Decreased activation of lateral orbitofrontal cortex during risky choices under uncertainty is associated with disadvantageous decision-making and suicidal behavior. *NeuroImage, 51*(3), 1275–1281. https://doi.org/10.1016/j.neuroimage.2010.03.027

Jones, C. J., Smith, H., & Llewellyn, C. (2014). Evaluating the effectiveness of health belief model interventions in improving adherence: A systematic review. *Health Psychology Review, 8*(3), 253–269. https://doi.org/10.1080/17437199.2013.802623

Kabat-Zinn, J. (2001). *Mindfulness meditation for everyday life.* Piatkus.

Kahler, C. W., Daughters, S. B., Leventhal, A. M., Gwaltney, C. J., & Palfai, T. P. (2007). Implicit associations between smoking and social consequences among smokers in cessation treatment. *Behaviour Research and Therapy, 45*(9), 2066–2077. https://doi.org/10.1016/j.brat.2007.03.004

Kahneman, D. (1999). Objective happiness. In D. Kahneman, E. Diener, & N. Schwarz (Eds.), *Well-being: Foundations of hedonic psychology* (pp. 3–25). Russell Sage Foundation.

Kahneman, D., Fredrickson, B. L., Schreiber, C. A., & Redelmeier, D. A. (1993). When more pain is preferred to less: Adding a better end. *Psychological Science, 4*(6), 401–405. https://doi.org/10.1111/j.1467-9280.1993.tb00589.x

Kahneman, D., & Tversky, A. (1979). Prospect theory: An analysis of decision under risk. *Econometrica*, *47*(2), 263–291. https://doi.org/10.2307/1914185

Kalsekar, I. D., Madhavan, S. S., Amonkar, M. M., Makela, E. H., Scott, V. G., Douglas, S. M., & Elswick, B. L. (2006). Depression in patients with Type 2 diabetes: Impact on adherence to oral hypoglycemic agents. *The Annals of Pharmacotherapy*, *40*(4), 605–611. https://doi.org/10.1345/aph.1G606

Kariis, H. M., Kasela, S., Jürgenson, T., Saar, A., Lass, J., Krebs, K., Võsa, U., Haan, E., Milani, L., Lehto, K., & the Estonian Biobank Research Team. (2023). The role of depression and antidepressant treatment in antihypertensive medication adherence and persistence: Utilising electronic health record data. *Journal of Psychiatric Research*, *168*, 269–278. https://doi.org/10.1016/j.jpsychires.2023.10.018

Kurdi, B., Seitchik, A. E., Axt, J. R., Carroll, T. J., Karapetyan, A., Kaushik, N., Tomezsko, D., Greenwald, A. G., & Banaji, M. R. (2019). Relationship between the Implicit Association Test and intergroup behavior: A meta-analysis. *American Psychologist*, *74*(5), 569–586. https://doi.org/10.1037/amp0000364

Lee, H. S., Addicott, M., Martin, L. E., Harris, K. J., Goggin, K., Richter, K. P., Patten, C. A., McClernon, F. J., Fleming, K., & Catley, D. (2018). Implicit attitudes and smoking behavior in a smoking cessation induction trial. *Nicotine & Tobacco Research*, *20*(1), 58–66. https://doi.org/10.1093/ntr/ntw259

Levin, E., & Levin, A. (2006). Evaluation of spoken dialogue technology for real-time health data collection. *Journal of Medical Internet Research*, *8*(4), Article e30. https://doi.org/10.2196/jmir.8.4.e30

Li, C., Lu, X., Xiao, J., & Chan, C. W. H. (2022). 'We can bear it!' Unpacking barriers to hepatocellular carcinoma screening among patients with hepatitis B: A qualitative study. *Journal of Clinical Nursing*, *31*(21–22), 3130–3143. https://doi.org/10.1111/jocn.16140

Liang, X., Zebrowitz, L. A., & Zhang, Y. (2010). Neural activation in the "reward circuit" shows a nonlinear response to facial attractiveness. *Social Neuroscience*, *5*(3), 320–334. https://doi.org/10.1080/17470911003619916

Lindenberg, S. (1985). Rational choice and sociological theory: New pressures on economics as a social science. *Journal of Institutional and Theoretical Economics*, *141*(2), 244–255.

Linehan, M. M. (1993). *Skills training manual for treatment of borderline personality disorder*. The Guilford Press.

Liu, L. L., & Park, D. C. (2004). Aging and medical adherence: The use of automatic processes to achieve effortful things. *Psychology and Aging*, *19*(2), 318–325. https://doi.org/10.1037/0882-7974.19.2.318

Liu, Q., Wang, H., Liu, A., Jiang, C., Li, W., Ma, H., & Geng, Q. (2022). Adherence to prescribed antihypertensive medication among patients with depression in the United States. *BMC Psychiatry*, *22*(1), 764. https://doi.org/10.1186/s12888-022-04424-x

Magai, C., Consedine, N., Neugut, A. I., & Hershman, D. L. (2007). Common psychosocial factors underlying breast cancer screening and breast cancer treatment adherence: A conceptual review and synthesis. *Journal of Women's Health*, *16*(1), 11–23. https://doi.org/10.1089/jwh.2006.0024

Magnan, R. E., Shorey Fennell, B. R., & Brady, J. M. (2017). Health decision making and behavior: The role of affect-laden constructs. *Social and Personality Psychology Compass*, *11*(8), Article e12333. https://doi.org/10.1111/spc3.12333

Mantler, T. (2013). A systematic review of smoking youths' perceptions of addiction and health risks associated with smoking: Utilizing the framework of the health belief model. *Addiction Research and Theory, 21*(4), 306–317. https://doi.org/10.3109/16066359.2012.727505

Marciniak, M. A., Shanahan, L., Rohde, J., Schulz, A., Wackerhagen, C., Kobylińska, D., Tuescher, O., Binder, H., Walter, H., Kalisch, R., & Kleim, B. (2020). Standalone smartphone cognitive behavioral therapy-based ecological momentary interventions to increase mental health: Narrative review. *JMIR mHealth and uHealth, 8*(11), Article e19836. https://doi.org/10.2196/19836

Mattavelli, S., Avishai, A., Perugini, M., Richetin, J., & Sheeran, P. (2017). How can implicit and explicit attitudes both be changed? Testing two interventions to promote consumption of green vegetables. *Annals of Behavioral Medicine, 51*(4), 511–518. https://doi.org/10.1007/s12160-016-9874-9

McEachan, R. R. C., Conner, M., Taylor, N. J., & Lawton, R. J. (2011). Prospective prediction of health-related behaviours with the theory of planned behaviour: A meta-analysis. *Health Psychology Review, 5*(2), 97–144. https://doi.org/10.1080/17437199.2010.521684

Mela, D. J. (2006). Novel food technologies: Enhancing appetite control in liquid meal replacers. *Obesity, 14*(S7), 179S–181S. https://doi.org/10.1038/oby.2006.302

Milne, S., Sheeran, P., & Orbell, S. (2000). Prediction and intervention in health-related behavior: A meta-analytic review of protection motivation theory. *Journal of Applied Social Psychology, 30*(1), 106–143. https://doi.org/10.1111/j.1559-1816.2000.tb02308.x

Moitra, E., LaPlante, A., Armstrong, M. L., Chan, P. A., & Stein, M. D. (2017). Pilot randomized controlled trial of acceptance-based behavior therapy to promote HIV acceptance, HIV disclosure, and retention in medical care. *AIDS and Behavior, 21*(9), 2641–2649. https://doi.org/10.1007/s10461-017-1780-z

Murphy, S. L., & Eaves, D. L. (2016). Exercising for the pleasure and for the pain of it: The implications of different forms of hedonistic thinking in theories of physical activity behavior. *Frontiers in Psychology, 7*, Article 843. https://doi.org/10.3389/fpsyg.2016.00843

Nabolsi, M. M., Wardam, L., & Al-Halabi, J. O. (2015). Quality of life, depression, adherence to treatment and illness perception of patients on haemodialysis. *International Journal of Nursing Practice, 21*(1), 1–10. https://doi.org/10.1111/ijn.12205

Naqvi, N. H., & Bechara, A. (2009, January). The hidden island of addiction: The insula. *Trends in Neurosciences, 32*(1), 56–67. https://doi.org/10.1016/j.tins.2008.09.009

Navarick, D. J. (2004). Analysis of impulsive choice: Assessing effects of implicit instructions. *The Psychological Record, 54*(4), 505–522. https://doi.org/10.1007/BF03395489

Nayok, S. B., Sreeraj, V. S., Shivakumar, V., & Venkatasubramanian, G. (2023). A primer on interoception and its importance in psychiatry. *Clinical Psychopharmacology and Neuroscience, 21*(2), 252–261. https://doi.org/10.9758/cpn.2023.21.2.252

Nicklas, L. B., Dunbar, M., & Wild, M. (2010). Adherence to pharmacological treatment of non-malignant chronic pain: The role of illness perceptions and medication beliefs. *Psychology & Health, 25*(5), 601–615. https://doi.org/10.1080/08870440902783610

Nock, M. K., Prinstein, M. J., & Sterba, S. K. (2009). Revealing the form and function of self-injurious thoughts and behaviors: A real-time ecological assessment study among adolescents and young adults. *Journal of Abnormal Psychology, 118*(4), 816–827. https://doi.org/10.1037/a0016948

O'Connor, M., Farrell, L., Munnelly, A., & McHugh, L. (2017). Citation analysis of relational frame theory: 2009–2016. *Journal of Contextual Behavioral Science, 6*(2), 152–158. https://doi.org/10.1016/j.jcbs.2017.04.009

O'Donohue, W. T., & Cucciare, M. A. (2005). Behavioral health economics and policy: An overview. In N. A. Cummings, W. T. O'Donohue, & M. A. Cucciare (Eds.), *Universal healthcare: Readings for mental health professionals* (pp. 19–45). Context Press.

Ogburn, D. F., Schoenbach, V. J., Edmonds, A., Pence, B. W., Powers, K. A., White, B. L., Dzialowy, N., & Samoff, E. (2019). Depression, ART adherence, and receipt of case management services by adults with HIV in North Carolina, medical monitoring project, 2009–2013. *AIDS and Behavior, 23*(4), 1004–1015. https://doi.org/10.1007/s10461-018-2365-1

Oh, H. S., Park, J. S., & Seo, W. S. (2013). Psychosocial influencers and mediators of treatment adherence in haemodialysis patients. *Journal of Advanced Nursing, 69*(9), 2041–2053. https://doi.org/10.1111/jan.12071

Olson, M. A., & Fazio, R. H. (2008). Implicit and explicit measures of attitudes: The perspective of the MODE model. In R. E. Petty, R. H. Fazio, & P. Briñol (Eds.), *Attitudes: Insights from the new implicit measures* (pp. 19–63). Psychology Press.

O'Malley, T. L., Krier, S. E., Bainbridge, M., Hawk, M. E., Egan, J. E., & Burke, J. G. (2023). Women's perspectives on barriers to potential PrEP uptake for HIV prevention: HIV risk assessment, relationship dynamics and stigma. *Culture, Health & Sexuality, 25*(6), 776–790. https://doi.org/10.1080/13691058.2022.2099016

Orbell, S., & Phillips, L. A. (2019). Automatic processes and self-regulation of illness. *Health Psychology Review, 13*(4), 378–405. https://doi.org/10.1080/17437199.2018.1503559

Pabst, S., Bertram, A., Zimmermann, T., Schiffer, M., & de Zwaan, M. (2015). Physician reported adherence to immunosuppressants in renal transplant patients: Prevalence, agreement, and correlates. *Journal of Psychosomatic Research, 79*(5), 364–371. https://doi.org/10.1016/j.jpsychores.2015.09.001

Park, C., Ma, X., Park, S. K., & Lawson, K. A. (2020). Association of depression with adherence to breast cancer screening among women aged 50 to 74 years in the United States. *Journal of Evaluation in Clinical Practice, 26*(6), 1677–1688. https://doi.org/10.1111/jep.13356

Parrinello, N., Napieralski, J., Gerlach, A. L., & Pohl, A. (2022). Embodied feelings—A meta-analysis on the relation of emotion intensity perception and interoceptive accuracy. *Physiology & Behavior, 254*, Article 113904. https://doi.org/10.1016/j.physbeh.2022.113904

Perski, O., Keller, J., Kale, D., Asare, B. Y.-A., Schneider, V., Powell, D., Naughton, F., Ten Hoor, G., Verboon, P., & Kwasnicka, D. (2022). Understanding health behaviours in context: A systematic review and meta-analysis of ecological momentary assessment studies of five key health behaviours. *Health Psychology Review, 16*(4), 576–601. https://doi.org/10.1080/17437199.2022.2112258

Perski, O., Kwasnicka, D., Kale, D., Schneider, V., Szinay, D., Ten Hoor, G., Asare, B. Y.-A., Verboon, P., Powell, D., Naughton, F., & Keller, J. (2023). Within-person associations between psychological and contextual factors and lapse incidence in smokers attempting to quit: A systematic review and meta-analysis of ecological momentary assessment studies. *Addiction, 118*(7), 1216–1231. https://doi.org/10.1111/add.16173

Pescosolido, B. A. (1992). Beyond rational choice: The social dynamics of how people seek help. *American Journal of Sociology, 97*(4), 1096–1138. https://doi.org/10.1086/229863

Plotnikoff, R. C., Costigan, S. A., Karunamuni, N., & Lubans, D. R. (2013). Social cognitive theories used to explain physical activity behavior in adolescents: A systematic review and meta-analysis. *Preventive Medicine, 56*(5), 245–253. https://doi.org/10.1016/j.ypmed.2013.01.013

Prince, S. A., Cardilli, L., Reed, J. L., Saunders, T. J., Kite, C., Douillette, K., Fournier, K., & Buckley, J. P. (2020). A comparison of self-reported and device measured sedentary behaviour in adults: A systematic review and meta-analysis. *The International Journal of Behavioral Nutrition and Physical Activity, 17*(1), 31–31. https://doi.org/10.1186/s12966-020-00938-3

Raaymakers, C., Garcia, Y., Cunningham, K., Krank, L., & Nemer-Kaiser, L. (2019). A systematic review of derived verbal behavior research. *Journal of Contextual Behavioral Science, 12*, 128–148. https://doi.org/10.1016/j.jcbs.2019.02.006

Ragin, D. F., Hussein, Y. M., Fichera, A., & Awai, J. (2020). Applying theories in health psychology. In D. F. Ragin & J. Keenan (Eds.), *Handbook of research methods in health psychology* (pp. 3–19). Routledge. https://doi.org/10.4324/9780429488320-2

Ramirez, J. J., Lee, C. M., Rhew, I. C., Olin, C. C., Abdallah, D. A., & Lindgren, K. P. (2020). What's the harm in getting high? Evaluating associations between marijuana and harm as predictors of concurrent and prospective marijuana use and misuse. *Journal of Studies on Alcohol and Drugs, 81*(1), 81–88. https://doi.org/10.15288/jsad.2020.81.81

Redelmeier, D. A., & Kahneman, D. (1996). Patients' memories of painful medical treatments: Real-time and retrospective evaluations of two minimally invasive procedures. *Pain, 66*(1), 3–8. https://doi.org/10.1016/0304-3959(96)02994-6

Redelmeier, D. A., Katz, J., & Kahneman, D. (2003). Memories of colonoscopy: A randomized trial. *Pain, 104*(1), 187–194. https://doi.org/10.1016/S0304-3959(03)00003-4

Reynolds, L. M., Consedine, N. S., & McCambridge, S. A. (2014). Mindfulness and disgust in colorectal cancer scenarios: Non-judging and non-reacting components predict avoidance when it makes sense. *Mindfulness, 5*(4), 442–452. https://doi.org/10.1007/s12671-013-0200-3

Ritchie, D., Van den Broucke, S., & Van Hal, G. (2021). The health belief model and theory of planned behavior applied to mammography screening: A systematic review and meta-analysis. *Public Health Nursing, 38*(3), 482–492. https://doi.org/10.1111/phn.12842

Rodríguez-Blanco, L., Carballo, J. J., & Baca-García, E. (2018). Use of ecological momentary assessment (EMA) in non-suicidal self-injury (NSSI): A systematic review. *Psychiatry Research, 263*, 212–219. https://doi.org/10.1016/j.psychres.2018.02.051

Rogers, R. W. (1983). Cognitive and physiological processes in fear appeals and attitude change: A revised theory of protection motivation. In J. T. Cacioppo &

R. E. Petty (Eds.), *Social psychophysiology: A sourcebook* (pp. 153–146). The Guilford Press.

Rosenstock, I. M. (1966). Why people use health services. *The Milbank Memorial Fund Quarterly, 44*(3), 94–127. https://doi.org/10.2307/3348967

Rosenstock, I. M. (1974). Historical origins of the health belief model. *Health Education Monographs, 2*(4), 328–335. https://doi.org/10.1177/109019817400200403

Rüsch, N., Todd, A. R., Bodenhausen, G. V., Weiden, P. J., & Corrigan, P. W. (2009). Implicit versus explicit attitudes toward psychiatric medication: Implications for insight and treatment adherence. *Schizophrenia Research, 112*(1–3), 119–122. https://doi.org/10.1016/j.schres.2009.04.011

Schick, A., Rauschenberg, C., Ader, L., Daemen, M., Wieland, L. M., Paetzold, I., Postma, M. R., Schulte-Strathaus, J. C. C., & Reininghaus, U. (2023). Novel digital methods for gathering intensive time series data in mental health research: Scoping review of a rapidly evolving field. *Psychological Medicine, 53*(1), 55–65. https://doi.org/10.1017/S0033291722003336

Schwartz, L. P., & Hursh, S. R. (2023). Time cost and demand: Implications for public policy. *Perspectives on Behavior Science, 46*(1), 51–66. https://doi.org/10.1007/s40614-022-00349-8

Scott-Sheldon, L. A. J. (2006). *Implicit–explicit ambivalent attitudes and health behaviors* (Publication No. 3221568) [Doctoral dissertation, University of Connecticut]. ProQuest Dissertations and Theses Global.

Sheeran, P., Gollwitzer, P. M., & Bargh, J. A. (2013). Nonconscious processes and health. *Health Psychology, 32*(5), 460–473. https://doi.org/10.1037/a0029203

Sheeran, P., Maki, A., Montanaro, E., Avishai-Yitshak, A., Bryan, A., Klein, W. M. P., Miles, E., & Rothman, A. J. (2016). The impact of changing attitudes, norms, and self-efficacy on health-related intentions and behavior: A meta-analysis. *Health Psychology, 35*(11), 1178–1188. https://doi.org/10.1037/hea0000387

Shiffman, S., & Kirchner, T. R. (2009). Cigarette-by-cigarette satisfaction during ad libitum smoking. *Journal of Abnormal Psychology, 118*(2), 348–359. https://doi.org/10.1037/a0015620

Shiffman, S., Stone, A. A., & Hufford, M. R. (2008). Ecological momentary assessment. *Annual Review of Clinical Psychology, 4*(1), 1–32. https://doi.org/10.1146/annurev.clinpsy.3.022806.091415

Shiffman, S., & Terhorst, L. (2017). Intermittent and daily smokers' subjective responses to smoking. *Psychopharmacology, 234*(19), 2911–2917. https://doi.org/10.1007/s00213-017-4682-x

Simon, H. A. (1955). A behavioral model of rational choice. *The Quarterly Journal of Economics, 69*(1), 99–118. https://doi.org/10.2307/1884852

Skinner, B. F. (1953). *Science and human behavior*. Macmillan.

Smith, S. G., Ellison, R., Hall, L., Clark, J., Hartley, S., Mason, E., Metherell, J., Olivier, C., Napp, V., Naik, J., Buckley, S., Hirst, C., Hartup, S., Neal, R. D., Velikova, G., Farrin, A., Collinson, M., & Graham, C. D. (2022). Acceptance and commitment therapy to support medication decision-making and quality of life in women with breast cancer: Protocol for a pilot randomised controlled trial. *Pilot and Feasibility Studies, 8*(1), 33–33. https://doi.org/10.1186/s40814-022-00985-6

Smith, S. G., Green, S. M. C., Ellison, R., Foy, R., Graham, C. D., Mason, E., French, D. P., Hall, L. H., Wilkes, H., McNaught, E., Raine, E., Walwyn, R., Howdon, D., Clark, J., Rousseau, N., Buxton, J., Moore, S. J. L., Parbutt, C., Velikova, G., . . .

Collinson, M. (2023). Refining and optimising a behavioural intervention to support endocrine therapy adherence (ROSETA) in UK women with breast cancer: Protocol for a pilot fractional factorial trial. *BMJ Open, 13*(2), e069971. https://doi.org/10.1136/bmjopen-2022-069971

Sritharan, R., & Gawronski, B. (2010). Changing implicit and explicit prejudice: Insights from the associative-propositional evaluation model. *Social Psychology, 41*(3), 113–123. https://doi.org/10.1027/1864-9335/a000017

Stevens, A., Peschk, I., & Schwarz, J. (2007). Implicit learning, executive function and hedonic activity in chronic polydrug abusers, currently abstinent polydrug abusers and controls. *Addiction, 102*(6), 937–946. https://doi.org/10.1111/j.1360-0443.2007.01823.x

Stroebe, W. (2022). The goal conflict model: A theory of the hedonic regulation of eating behavior. *Current Opinion in Behavioral Sciences, 48*, Article 101203. https://doi.org/10.1016/j.cobeha.2022.101203

Stroebe, W., & Stroebe, M. (1995). *Social psychology and health*. Brooks/Cole Publishing.

Swendsen, J., Ben-Zeev, D., & Granholm, E. (2011). Real-time electronic ambulatory monitoring of substance use and symptom expression in schizophrenia. *The American Journal of Psychiatry, 168*(2), 202–209. https://doi.org/10.1176/appi.ajp.2010.10030463

Taflinger, S., & Sattler, S. (2024). A situational test of the health belief model: How perceived susceptibility mediates the effects of the environment on behavioral intentions. *Social Science & Medicine, 346*, Article 116715. https://doi.org/10.1016/j.socscimed.2024.116715

Tao, J., Vermund, S. H., & Qian, H.-Z. (2018). Association between depression and antiretroviral therapy use among people living with HIV: A meta-analysis. *AIDS and Behavior, 22*(5), 1542–1550. https://doi.org/10.1007/s10461-017-1776-8

Tavakoli, B., Feizi, A., Zamani-Alavijeh, F., & Shahnazi, H. (2024). Factors influencing breast cancer screening practices among women worldwide: A systematic review of observational and qualitative studies. *BMC Women's Health, 24*(1), Article 268. https://doi.org/10.1186/s12905-024-03096-x

Thush, C., & Wiers, R. W. (2007). Explicit and implicit alcohol-related cognitions and the prediction of future drinking in adolescents. *Addictive Behaviors, 32*(7), 1367–1383. https://doi.org/10.1016/j.addbeh.2006.09.011

Tversky, A., & Kahneman, D. (1973). Availability: A heuristic for judging frequency and probability. *Cognitive Psychology, 5*(2), 207–232. https://doi.org/10.1016/0010-0285(73)90033-9

Volpp, K. G., Friedman, W., Romano, P. S., Rosen, A., & Silber, J. H. (2010). Residency training at a crossroads: Duty-hour standards 2010. *Annals of Internal Medicine, 153*(12), 826–828. https://doi.org/10.7326/0003-4819-153-12-201012210-00287

Waters, A. J., Carter, B. L., Robinson, J. D., Wetter, D. W., Lam, C. Y., & Cinciripini, P. M. (2007). Implicit attitudes to smoking are associated with craving and dependence. *Drug and Alcohol Dependence, 91*(2–3), 178–186. https://doi.org/10.1016/j.drugalcdep.2007.05.024

Wiers, R. W., Rinck, M., Kordts, R., Houben, K., & Strack, F. (2010). Retraining automatic action-tendencies to approach alcohol in hazardous drinkers. *Addiction, 105*(2), 279–287. https://doi.org/10.1111/j.1360-0443.2009.02775.x

Williams, D. M. (2008). Exercise, affect, and adherence: An integrated model and a case for self-paced exercise. *Journal of Sport & Exercise Psychology, 30*(5), 471–496. https://doi.org/10.1123/jsep.30.5.471

Williams, D. M., & Evans, D. R. (2014). Current emotion research in health behavior science. *Emotion Review, 6*(3), 277–287. https://doi.org/10.1177/1754073914523052

Willis, J., & Todorov, A. (2006). First impressions: Making up your mind after a 100-ms exposure to a face. *Psychological Science, 17*(7), 592–598. https://doi.org/10.1111/j.1467-9280.2006.01750.x

Winston, J. S., Strange, B. A., O'Doherty, J., & Dolan, R. J. (2002). Automatic and intentional brain responses during evaluation of trustworthiness of faces. *Nature Neuroscience, 5*(3), 277–283. https://doi.org/10.1038/nn816

Wood, R. Y., & Della-Monica, N. R. (2015). Breast cancer threat appraisal: Design and psychometric analysis of a new scale for older women. *International Journal of Older People Nursing, 10*(2), 94–104. https://doi.org/10.1111/opn.12054

3 DECISION MAKING AND SOCIAL MARGINALIZATION

SAI SNIGDHA TALLURI AND YEN CHUN TSENG

The implementation and effectiveness of shared decision making (SDM) is profoundly affected by social determinants, such as economic stability, education, access to health care, and immigration. Further, personal identities, including ethnicity, gender identity, and sexual orientation can shape individual experiences, preferences, and engagement in the decision-making process. Thus, understanding how these factors play into SDM is crucial for developing inclusive and effective decision-making practices. This chapter explores how social determinants and personal identities affect SDM and draws on evidence to highlight the complexities and potential strategies to address these challenges.

SHARED DECISION MAKING AND SOCIODEMOGRAPHIC FACTORS

Evidence about how race, ethnicity, gender identity, and sexual orientation affect SDM for people with serious mental illness (SMI) is limited. Therefore, this section aims to explore how these identities affect SDM in health care

https://doi.org/10.1037/0000478-003
Shared Decision Making and Serious Mental Illness, P. W. Corrigan (Editor)

settings and discusses how lessons learned can be applied to individuals with SDM.

Race and Ethnicity

Disparities in communication and SDM are well documented among ethnic groups. Research has shown that physician communication and decision making are influenced by racial and ethnic differences between physicians and patients (Alkhamees & Alasqah, 2023; Shen et al., 2019; van Ryn & Burke, 2000). In the Medical Outcomes Study, patients of color rated their physicians' decision-making styles as less participatory than did White patients (Kaplan et al., 1995). Specifically, African Americans and others in ethnicity-discordant relationships with their providers reported less involvement in medical decisions and less partnership with providers (Cooper-Patrick et al., 1999; Kaplan et al., 1995). One study on physician–patient communication that directly addressed the issue of ethnicity demonstrated that physicians used better questioning and facilitating skills and empathy skills with White American patients compared with Spanish American patients (Hooper et al., 1982).

A number of factors can account for these problems. Health care providers may be influenced by implicit racial and ethnic stereotypes while interpreting symptoms, individual behavior, and decision making (Schulman et al., 1999). These implicit attitudes may be expressed in different ways, including using a dominant and condescending tone when talking to patients, being less thorough with diagnostic work, and not providing interpreters when required (Hall et al., 2015). Providers may also make patients of color wait longer for assessment or treatment or spend less time with them than their White counterparts. These behaviors decrease the likelihood that patients will feel heard and valued by their providers, thus resulting in decreased motivation to engage in SDM.

Providers' preconceived beliefs about who is more likely to prefer an active role may influence how they engage different ethnic groups in decision making (Peek et al., 2010). When compared with White patients, some White providers view African American patients as less intelligent, less able to adhere to treatment regimens, and more likely to engage in risky health behaviors (van Ryn & Burke, 2000). As a result, African Americans health care visits are less participatory, and providers are more verbally dominant, deliver less information, and communicate in less person-centered ways than with White patients (Epstein et al., 1985; Johnson et al., 2004). Indeed, Ge et al. (2009) videotaped physician and patient consultations and found that

White physicians had largely one-sided conversations with Chinese, Hispanic, and African American patients. They observed that physicians did most of the talking and rarely solicited questions from patients of color. Further, providers may lack understanding of individuals' ethnic and cultural disease models or attribution of symptoms. For instance, research has suggested that health care providers may be more paternalistic with Hispanic individuals when it comes to decision making, perhaps related to language barriers or unfamiliarity with cultural differences and expectations (Cooper-Patrick et al., 1999).

Other factors might contribute to decision making being less of a shared endeavor during visits, including language barriers, low health literacy and educational status, and lack of self-efficacy regarding managing one's health (Durand et al., 2014; Seo et al., 2016; Toapanta et al., 2023). To be effective, SDM requires a certain level of health literacy, which may be lower in individuals from ethnic minority groups. For instance, two thirds of Hispanic Americans have limited health literacy skills and hence have greater difficulty understanding interactions with health care providers (Greenberg & Paulsen, 2006). In addition to health literacy, individuals from ethnic minority groups who have difficulty with English are less likely than White people who have difficulty with English to generate empathy from and establish rapport with physicians; they also are less likely to receive pertinent information or to be encouraged to engage in SDM (Ferguson & Candib, 2002). When providers encounter individuals with low health literacy, they are often tempted to make decisions for them, which reinforces those individuals' passive role (Coulter & Collins, 2011).

Trust is one mechanism by which SDM can influence treatment outcomes. Mistrust of the physician is also a mechanism by which ethnicity and other differences may influence SDM (Kraetschmer et al., 2004). Alvidrez et al. (2008) highlighted that stigma and historical mistrust significantly reduces service use among African Americans, which makes it challenging to establish effective SDM processes. Mistrust between providers and patients of color also occurs because of barriers to cross-cultural communication, racism, and impersonal patient relationships with providers.

Sexual Orientation and Gender Identity

The term *sexual and gender minorities* (SGMs) describes individuals whose sexual orientation, gender identity, or gender expression is different from the majority. SGMs distrust their health care providers and the health care system in general (Kaiser Family Foundation, 2024), which can act as a barrier to SDM. Growing research has suggested that SGMs who belong to minority racial and ethnic groups may face more complicated challenges while doing SDM than White SGMs. For instance, research has suggested that, for SGMs, there is evidence that providers' unconscious ethnic or heterosexual biases can influence medical care and their expectations for patient adherence and SDM engagement (Peek et al., 2016). Insufficient knowledge of SGMs' life experiences and health needs limits the effective exchange of health care information during the SDM process (Johnson et al., 2004).

Sexual and gender minority (SGM) group members may also anticipate negative experiences with health care providers and thus may frequently delay or avoid seeking care (Mail, 2002). Researchers found that 15% of individuals who identified as SGM reported that they were fearful about accessing health care services outside the SGM community, and 13% reported that they were denied health care services or provided with subpar care as a result of their sexual orientation or gender identity (Fredriksen-Goldsen et al., 2014). Those who do seek care often do not feel comfortable disclosing their sexual orientation or gender identity, which prevents them from having open and honest communication about their health care needs and preferences, further impeding SDM (Chin et al., 2016).

Age

Some literature has discussed the association between age and SDM for people with severe mental illness. One cross-sectional study of psychiatric outpatients in Spain found that with increasing age, patients felt less involved in SDM (De las Cuevas & Peñate, 2014). Another European multicenter study found that providers more frequently adopted SDM when their patients were younger (Luciano et al., 2020). In terms of preferences for SDM and age, results have been conflicting. A few studies concluded that compared with older adults, younger adults prefer to participate in SDM (Hill & Laugharne, 2006; Say et al., 2006), whereas other studies suggested that older adults prefer involvement (Say et al., 2006). Other research has suggested that age has no effect on decision making (Park et al., 2014; Wright-Berryman & Kim, 2016). These differences in findings can be attributed to a number of factors, including lack of consensus on what constitutes an "older person" (Burns et al., 2021). Nonetheless, older adults with mental health conditions face specific barriers that may hinder participation in SDM. These include difficulties in communication, such as hearing loss, speech impediments, and reduced cognitive processing speed (Bynum et al., 2014).

Shared Decision Making and Sociodemographic Factors in Serious Mental Illness

The literature on the associations between demographic factors and SDM for people with SMI is inadequate. One study used the Shared Decision-Making Scale (Salyers et al., 2012) to evaluate transcripts of visits at community mental health centers and found that demographic characteristics of service users and providers, such as age, gender, and race, were not significantly associated with SDM scores (Fukui et al., 2014). Another similar study evaluated SDM during medication management visits and established that overall SDM was not associated with any demographic characteristics. Additionally, a recent scoping review examined associations between patient-related characteristics and SDM in the context of physical and mental health care (Keij et al., 2022). The authors found that, in more than half the studies, there was no significant associations between age, gender, and SDM. Further research is needed to determine which patient characteristics might be associated with SDM for people with SMI.

SHARED DECISION MAKING AND SOCIAL DISADVANTAGE

Individuals with SMI face numerous social disadvantages, such as high rates of unemployment and poverty; decreased educational attainment; lack of access to health care; and increased homelessness, morbidity and mortality, social isolation, and involvement with the criminal justice system both as victims and arrestees (Alegría et al., 2018). In general, disadvantaged groups have difficulty accessing relevant services and actively engaging in health care (Durand et al., 2014). These disparities significantly affect an individual's ability to access and benefit from SDM.

Socioeconomic Status

Many people with SMI are undereducated and underemployed and have high rates of poverty when compared with the general population (Corrigan et al., 2014; McAlpine & Alang, 2021). Living in poverty means that people with SMI may not have access to services that prioritize SDM, may lack the means to pay for health care services, or may not qualify for insurance or benefits that would offset the cost of services that include SDM. People living in poverty are less likely to live in geographic areas with health care resources, such as SDM. Even when SDM is available for individuals from lower socioeconomic status (SES) backgrounds, people often reported feeling less involved in medical decision making compared with those from higher SES backgrounds. They cited barriers such as time constraints, perceived power imbalances, and lack of understanding (Peek et al., 2010).

Criminal Justice Involvement

People with SMI are also involved in the criminal justice system both as arrestees and victims at high rates (Anderson et al., 2015). People with SMI who are arrested face considerable stigma, including perceptions of dangerousness, violence, and dishonesty (Adekson, 2018; Pescosolido et al., 2019; Rade et al., 2018). Although people who work in corrections settings endorse lower negative attitudes toward people with SMI (Lowder et al., 2019; Matejkowski et al., 2010), stigma can still be a barrier to SDM in this context. For example, a survey among community corrections officers aimed at identifying predictors of attitudes supportive of SDM found that stigma toward people with SMI had the strongest relationship with attitudes supportive of SDM. In other words, officers who viewed people with SMI as fundamentally different from supervisors or as too sick to collaborate in supervision planning were less likely to support SDM (Matejkowski & Severson, 2020).

Providers who wish to engage victims of crime with SMI in SDM must use a trauma-informed approach and work on creating a safe and supportive environment that is based on trust. SDM can help victims regain a sense of autonomy by involving them in decisions about their care. SDM can also help victims of crime feel empowered as providers offer different treatment choices and respect the individual's preferences.

Immigration Status

People with SMI who have migrated from outside the United States may experience issues resulting from their immigration and acculturation status that can affect health care decision making. Individuals who are undocumented may fear deportation, not wanting to disclose immigration status when seeking services. Other factors related to immigration that can affect SDM include being unable to take time off to work to attend medical appointments, struggling to access immigrant-friendly services or referrals, and facing difficulties meeting paperwork requirements because of a lack of proper identification or proof of income (Dang et al., 2012; Morales, 2013; Viruell-Fuentes et al., 2012). Similar to issues with patients of different ethnicities, individuals who have migrated from outside the United States may have different health and illness beliefs than their providers and have low health literacy (Dobler et al., 2017).

INTERSECTIONALITY

Although there is growing literature about SDM among various groups of individuals, little is known about these issues among populations that live at the intersection of such identities. The term *intersectionality* was coined by Kimberlé Crenshaw (1989) to explain the racism and sexism faced by African American women. This term has since been expanded to describe how race, ethnicity, gender, and other characteristics intersect with one another to create distinct experiences of marginalization and privilege. Intersectionality emphasizes how people who are members of multiple marginalized groups or with multiple disadvantages can experience interactive effects on their health and well-being. Individuals who have multiple disadvantaged identities are more likely to report interpersonal discrimination, microaggressions, psychological distress, worse self-rated health, and more functional limitations than their singly disadvantaged counterparts (Denise, 2014).

People with SMI are members of numerous social groups with different languages of origin, culture, SES, faith, family structure, and health needs. People with SMI who identify as ethnic minorities or SGMs can be disadvantaged within multiple social systems and identities. To engage patients in SDM, providers need to acknowledge the uniqueness of individual identities and take into consideration the complex interactions among these identities (Ng, 2016). A growing body of evidence has suggested that intersections of race, ethnicity, gender identity, and sexual orientation affect access to care, health risk profiles, and health outcomes. However, individuals who are members of both ethnic minority groups and SGMs are often overlooked in research. The case example of Alex (see Exhibit 3.1) highlights the barriers to SDM.

Latine SGMs are affected by key intersectional issues, including lack of effective SDM approaches to address diversity (e.g., immigration, acculturation, SES, ethnicity, language proficiency). Heterosexist and racist microaggressions experienced by people of color who identify as SGMs in clinical settings affect mental health, physical health, health-related behaviors, and service use (Ng, 2016). Consider, for example, a Latina woman with depression who goes to a clinic for a routine checkup. Without asking about her sexual orientation, the provider repeatedly asks questions about her husband or boyfriend. Further, the provider makes assumptions, asking,

EXHIBIT 3.1. Case Example: Alex

Alex is a 42-year-old, undocumented, cisgender Latina woman who identifies as queer. Alex has lived in the United States for 20 years but was born in Mexico. She is in a long-term relationship with a cisgender woman. However, Alex's family does not know about her relationship because she fears they would not approve. Alex has been diagnosed with major depressive disorder and has experienced multiple hospitalizations because of previous suicide attempts. Alex has been unable to find stable employment and currently resides with her partner in a one-bedroom apartment.

Alex has been referred to a community mental health clinic that emphasizes a shared decision making (SDM) approach in managing serious mental illness. Alex's psychiatrist is Dr. Smith, a 55-year-old, straight, White, cisgender woman. Alex did not disclose her sexual orientation to Dr. Smith for fear that she would out Alex to her community. Although Alex can speak and understand some English, she is mainly Spanish-speaking. Her psychiatrist, on the other hand, does not speak or understand Spanish, so their encounters are always in English, which makes it hard for Alex.

During one medication management appointment, the psychiatrist noticed bruises on Alex's arms. The psychiatrist questioned Alex, who reluctantly admitted that her partner is physically abusive but that she is afraid to end their relationship because she has nowhere else to go. Alex's psychiatrist provided her with phone numbers of local domestic violence shelters and referred her to a social worker. Dr. Smith was unaware that Alex feared that if she sought services or contacted the domestic violence shelter, she might run into legal problems because of her undocumented status. Dr. Smith ended the appointment without scheduling a follow-up appointment.

This case illustrates ways that multiple minority identities, such as ethnicity, immigration status, sexual orientation, cultural norms, and heteronormativity, intersect and act as barriers to SDM. Alex was also unwilling to disclose her sexual orientation and immigration status because of stigma, family expectations, and cultural norms that place emphasis on the family rather than the individual. In terms of SDM, the provider did not consult with Alex before making a referral; instead, Alex's psychiatrist referred Alex to a domestic violence shelter, where Alex feared that she might have to disclose her immigration status.

Note. Case examples in this book are hypothetical.

"Where are you really from?" implying that the patient is an outsider. Unfortunately, many providers lack the experience required to address issues at the intersection of multiple identities.

To address the unique issues faced by individuals with intersecting identities, providers must appreciate the heterogeneity of SGM racial/ethnic patients. They can do this by listening attentively and without judgment to patients about their specific health care needs and by considering their values, preferences, and beliefs so that they can form a patient–provider relationship based on trust, respect, and understanding. This, in turn, can facilitate information sharing and open and effective communication as well as empower patients to engage in SDM and participate actively in the decision-making process. For instance, in the case of Alex, her provider missed opportunities to empower Alex to engage in SDM because the provider did not establish a trusting relationship with Alex. However, every patient's desire to engage in SDM is likely to be different, and providers must respect these limits (Ng, 2016). For example, while selecting a particular drug to treat diabetes, many patients might defer to their provider's judgment, whereas some might prefer to understand the benefits, risks, and side effects of each option before making their own decision.

Providers caring for individuals who are members of ethnic and SGM groups can incorporate an intersectional lens in SDM by establishing a safe environment. Key to this effort is using the correct terminology (e.g., pronouns, preferred name) and providing materials in different languages or ensuring access to medical interpreters. The idea of cultural competency has been recognized as an integral part of patient care; most often, culture is assumed to refer to race, ethnicity, or religion. A broader interpretation of cultural competence includes many other characteristics discussed in this section. Additionally, culture is now perceived as a fluid subjective characteristic that changes because the individual may feel they belong to different cultures. Hence, the concept of cultural humility may be a skill that providers should strive to attain. Cultural humility training for providers can improve their ability to communicate with diverse patients and engage them in SDM. Instead of programs that teach providers broadly about ethnic, racial, or SGM groups, programs in which providers are taught to be aware of biases and stereotypes may be more effective (Crenshaw, 2010; Kleinman & Benson, 2006; Seeleman et al., 2009). Providers can also be curious about individual identities and beliefs that influence health care decision making.

ENHANCING SHARED DECISION MAKING BY ADDRESSING SOCIAL DETERMINANTS

One way to enhance SDM is by promoting cultural competence of providers. Proponents of cultural competence and humility have suggested that, to engage people from different ethnic groups, providers need to possess flexible skills. These skills can be imparted through wide array of training approaches, including cultural awareness, definitions of cultural and linguistic competency, communication skills, and health care–specific teachings.

Research has reported several provider-level and patient-level factors that can enhance the SDM experience for patients of color and SGMs (Jolles et al., 2019). Provider-level actions include explanations of changes in health screening guidelines, disclosure of harms and side effects of treatment options, willingness to consider patient preferences, and the fostering of a warm and personal relationship with patients. Patient-level factors include participation in interventions to build conference, assertiveness, and self-efficacy; disclosure of use of complementary health approaches; readiness to make decisions; and concordance on an SDM approach with the provider. Referring to the case example of Alex, her psychiatrist, Dr. Smith, could have facilitated SDM by hiring an interpreter to help foster a warm and personal relationship with Alex.

Another way of increasing SDM among individuals affected by social and systemic disadvantages is to look beyond the patient–provider relationship and focus on the context in which services are provided. DeMeester and colleagues (2016) proposed a conceptual model for how organizations can restructure their practices to support SDM among minorities. In this model, clinician and individual activation can be improved through six organizational drivers—(a) workflow procedures, (b) health information technology, (c) organizational structure and culture, (d) resources or the clinic environment, (e) training and education, and (f) incentives or disincentives—that act through four mechanisms: (a) continuity and coordination; (b) ease of SDM; (c) knowledge and skills; and (d) attitudes and beliefs, all of which improve clinician and patient activation of SDM. Together, the drivers and mechanisms lead to *activation*, which is when clinicians and individuals have the knowledge, skills, and motivation to engage in SDM.

Consider, for example, the *health information technology driver*, which refers to any technology that supports SDM, such as electronic medical records (EMRs). There is great potential for EMRs to support SDM if, for example, only labels and names chosen by the individual are recorded in the EMR, documenting an individual's identity only in ways with which they feel comfortable (Gay and Lesbian Medical Association, 2006). Another example is if organizations choose to use EMRs that capture data on key aspects of a person's identity, such as race, ethnicity, sexual orientation, gender identity, and preferred names or pronouns (Institute of Medicine, 2011). Out of these four mechanisms, the health information technology driver likely affects SDM through continuity and coordination and knowledge and skills. In other words, improving health information technology can lead to better coordination across team members and visits and can also help providers individualize care and elicit patient preferences, values, and beliefs.

Another way of addressing social determinants and enhancing SDM includes a model, labeled "the environment" that was developed based on SDM among African Americans and intersectionality (Peek et al., 2016). In this model, the environment includes both physical (e.g., resources, location, infrastructure) and social contexts (e.g., culture, religion, politics) that shape individuals' experiences and expectations of health systems and physician interactions. Specifically, the model hypothesizes that social identity, structural inequalities, and past experiences and beliefs about physicians and health care delivery all affect SDM. In addition, this model also includes interactions within patients' health care environment and communications with their physician, which allows for the examination of more intersectional factors. For instance, when individuals perceive racism or heterosexism from a provider, they may alter their behavior to influence provider perceptions and ensure that they receive high quality care. The use of such impression management strategies can influence the patient–provider relationship and, in turn, SDM.

CONCLUSION

Sociodemographic factors and social disadvantages can impede SDM for people with SMI. Little is known about SDM among those who identify as ethnic minorities and SGMs. Understanding how these factors can be addressed to improve SDM among ethnic minorities and SGMs is an important step in addressing health disparities. Much of the research on enhancing SDM is focused on improving the provider–patient relationship; however, more recent models suggest focusing on the context in which services are provided, such as the organization where SDM takes place, social context, and individual experience. These models do not take SMI into consideration; thus, there is a need to develop new models that consider people with SMI.

REFERENCES

Adekson, B. (2018). *Supervision and treatment experiences of probationers with mental illness: Analyses of contemporary issues in community corrections*. Routledge. https://doi.org/10.4324/9781315180410

Alegría, M., NeMoyer, A., Falgàs Bagué, I., Wang, Y., & Alvarez, K. (2018). Social determinants of mental health: Where we are and where we need to go. *Current Psychiatry Reports, 20*(11), Article 95. https://doi.org/10.1007/s11920-018-0969-9

Alkhamees, M., & Alasqah, I. (2023). Patient–physician communication in intercultural settings: An integrative review. *Heliyon, 9*(12), Article e22667. https://doi.org/10.1016/j.heliyon.2023.e22667

Alvidrez, J., Snowden, L. R., & Kaiser, D. M. (2008). The experience of stigma among Black mental health consumers. *Journal of Health Care for the Poor and Underserved, 19*(3), 874–893. https://doi.org/10.1353/hpu.0.0058

Anderson, A., von Esenwein, S., Spaulding, A., & Druss, B. (2015). Involvement in the criminal justice system among attendees of an urban mental health center. *Health & Justice, 3*(1), Article 4. https://doi.org/10.1186/s40352-015-0017-3

Burns, L., da Silva, A. L., & John, A. (2021). Shared decision-making preferences in mental health: Does age matter? A systematic review. *Journal of Mental Health, 30*(5), 634–645. https://doi.org/10.1080/09638237.2020.1793124

Bynum, J. P. W., Barre, L., Reed, C., & Passow, H. (2014). Participation of very old adults in health care decisions. *Medical Decision Making, 34*(2), 216–230. https://doi.org/10.1177/0272989X13508008

Chin, M. H., Lopez, F. Y., Nathan, A. G., & Cook, S. C. (2016). Improving shared decision making with LGBT racial and ethnic minority patients. *Journal of General Internal Medicine, 31*(6), 591–593. https://doi.org/10.1007/s11606-016-3607-4

Cooper-Patrick, L., Gallo, J. J., Gonzales, J. J., Vu, H. T., Powe, N. R., Nelson, C., & Ford, D. E. (1999). Race, gender, and partnership in the patient–physician relationship. *JAMA, 282*(6), 583–589. https://doi.org/10.1001/jama.282.6.583

Corrigan, P. W., Pickett, S., Batia, K., & Michaels, P. J. (2014). Peer navigators and integrated care to address ethnic health disparities of people with serious mental illness. *Social Work in Public Health, 29*(6), 581–593. https://doi.org/10.1080/19371918.2014.893854

Coulter, A., & Collins, A. (2011). *Making shared decision-making a reality: No decision about me, without me.* The King's Fund.

Crenshaw, K. (1989). Demarginalizing the intersection of race and sex: A Black feminist critique of antidiscrimination doctrine, feminist theory and antiracist politics. *University of Chicago Legal Forum, 1989*, Article 8. https://chicagounbound.uchicago.edu/uclf/vol1989/iss1/8

Crenshaw, K. W. (2010). Twenty years of critical race theory: Looking back to move forward. *Connecticut Law Review, 43*(5), Article 1253.

Dang, B. N., Giordano, T. P., & Kim, J. H. (2012). Sociocultural and structural barriers to care among undocumented Latino immigrants with HIV infection. *Journal of Immigrant and Minority Health, 14*(1), 124–131. https://doi.org/10.1007/s10903-011-9542-x

De las Cuevas, C., & Peñate, W. (2014). Preferences for participation in shared decision making of psychiatric outpatients with affective disorders. *Open Journal of Psychiatry, 4*(1), 16–23. https://doi.org/10.4236/ojpsych.2014.41004

DeMeester, R. H., Lopez, F. Y., Moore, J. E., Cook, S. C., & Chin, M. H. (2016). A model of organizational context and shared decision making: Application to LGBT racial and ethnic minority patients. *Journal of General Internal Medicine, 31*, 651–662. https://doi.org/10.1007/s11606-016-3608-3

Denise, E. J. (2014). Multiple disadvantaged statuses and health: The role of multiple forms of discrimination. *Journal of Health and Social Behavior, 55*(1), 3–19. https://doi.org/10.1177/0022146514521215

Dobler, C. C., Spencer-Bonilla, G., Gionfriddo, M. R., & Brito, J. P. (2017). Shared decision making in immigrant patients. *Cureus, 9*(7), Article e1461. https://doi.org/10.7759/cureus.146

Durand, M.-A., Carpenter, L., Dolan, H., Bravo, P., Mann, M., Bunn, F., & Elwyn, G. (2014). Do interventions designed to support shared decision-making reduce health inequalities? A systematic review and meta-analysis. *PLOS ONE, 9*(4), Article e94670. https://doi.org/10.1371/journal.pone.0094670

Epstein, A. M., Taylor, W. C., & Seage, G. R., III. (1985). Effects of patients' socioeconomic status and physicians' training and practice on patient-doctor communication. *The American Journal of Medicine, 78*(1), 101–106. https://doi.org/10.1016/0002-9343(85)90469-3

Ferguson, W. J., & Candib, L. M. (2002). Culture, language, and the doctor–patient relationship. *Family Medicine, 34*(5), 353–361. https://www.stfm.org/FamilyMedicine/Vol34Issue5/Ferguson353

Fredriksen-Goldsen, K. I., Cook-Daniels, L., Kim, H.-J., Erosheva, E. A., Emlet, C. A., Hoy-Ellis, C. P., Goldsen, J., & Muraco, A. (2014). Physical and mental health of transgender older adults: An at-risk and underserved population. *The Gerontologist, 54*(3), 488–500. https://doi.org/10.1093/geront/gnt021

Fukui, S., Salyers, M. P., Matthias, M. S., Collins, L., Thompson, J., Coffman, M., & Torrey, W. C. (2014). Predictors of shared decision making and level of agreement between consumers and providers in psychiatric care. *Community Mental Health Journal, 50*(4), 375–382. https://doi.org/10.1007/s10597-012-9584-0

Gay and Lesbian Medical Association. (2006). *Guidelines for care of lesbian, gay, bisexual, and transgender patients.*

Ge, G., Burke, N., Somkin, C. P., & Pasick, R. (2009). Considering culture in physician–patient communication during colorectal cancer screening. *Qualitative Health Research, 19*(6), 778–789. https://doi.org/10.1177/1049732309335269

Greenberg, K., & Paulsen, J. (2006, September). *The health literacy of America's adults: Results from the 2003 National Assessment of Adult Literacy* (NCES Report No. 2006-483). U.S. Department of Education. https://nces.ed.gov/pubs2006/2006483.pdf

Hall, W. J., Chapman, M. V., Lee, K. M., Merino, Y. M., Thomas, T. W., Payne, B. K., Eng, E., Day, S. H., & Coyne-Beasley, T. (2015). Implicit racial/ethnic bias among health care professionals and its influence on health care outcomes: A systematic review. *American Journal of Public Health, 105*(12), e60–e76. https://doi.org/10.2105/AJPH.2015.302903

Hill, S. A., & Laugharne, R. (2006). Decision making and information seeking preferences among psychiatric patients. *Journal of Mental Health, 15*(1), 75–84. https://doi.org/10.1080/09638230500512250

Hooper, E. M., Comstock, L. M., Goodwin, J. M., & Goodwin, J. S. (1982). Patient characteristics that influence physician behavior. *Medical Care, 20*(6), 630–638. https://doi.org/10.1097/00005650-198206000-00009

Institute of Medicine. (2011). *The health of lesbian, gay, bisexual, and transgender (LGBT) people: Building a foundation for better understanding.* National Academies Press.

Johnson, R. L., Roter, D., Powe, N. R., & Cooper, L. A. (2004). Patient race/ethnicity and quality of patient-physician communication during medical visits. *American Journal of Public Health, 94*(12), 2084–2090. https://doi.org/10.2105/AJPH.94.12.2084

Jolles, M. P., Richmond, J., & Thomas, K. C. (2019). Minority patient preferences, barriers, and facilitators for shared decision-making with health care providers in the USA: A systematic review. *Patient Education and Counseling, 102*(7), 1251–1262. https://doi.org/10.1016/j.pec.2019.02.003

Kaiser Family Foundation. (2024, April 2). *LGBT adults' experiences with discrimination and health care disparities: Findings from the KFF Survey of Racism, Discrimination, and Health.* https://www.kff.org/racial-equity-and-health-policy/poll-finding/lgbt-adults-experiences-with-discrimination-and-health-care-disparities-findings-from-the-kff-survey-of-racism-discrimination-and-health/

Kaplan, S. H., Gandek, B., Greenfield, S., Rogers, W., & Ware, J. E. (1995). Patient and visit characteristics related to physicians' participatory decision-making style: Results from the Medical Outcomes Study. *Medical Care, 33*(12), 1176–1187. https://doi.org/10.1097/00005650-199512000-00002

Keij, S. M., de Boer, J. E., Stiggelbout, A. M., Bruine de Bruin, W., Peters, E., Moaddine, S., Kunneman, M., & Pieterse, A. H. (2022). How are patient-related characteristics associated with shared decision-making about treatment? A scoping review of quantitative studies. *BMJ Open, 12*(5), Article e057293. https://doi.org/10.1136/bmjopen-2021-057293

Kleinman, A., & Benson, P. (2006). Anthropology in the clinic: The problem of cultural competency and how to fix it. *PLOS Medicine, 3*(10), Article e294. https://doi.org/10.1371/journal.pmed.0030294

Kraetschmer, N., Sharpe, N., Urowitz, S., & Deber, R. B. (2004). How does trust affect patient preferences for participation in decision-making? *Health Expectations, 7*(4), 317–326. https://doi.org/10.1111/j.1369-7625.2004.00296.x

Lowder, E. M., Ray, B. R., & Gruenewald, J. A. (2019). Criminal justice professionals' attitudes toward mental illness and substance use. *Community Mental Health Journal, 55*(3), 428–439. https://doi.org/10.1007/s10597-019-00370-3

Luciano, M., Sampogna, G., Del Vecchio, V., Loos, S., Slade, M., Clarke, E., Nagy, M., Kovacs, A., Munk-Jørgensen, P., Krogsgaard Bording, M., Kawohl, W., Rössler, W., Puschner, B., Fiorillo, A., & the CEDAR Study Group. (2020). When does shared decision making is adopted in psychiatric clinical practice? Results from a European multicentric study. *European Archives of Psychiatry and Clinical Neuroscience, 270*(6), 645–653. https://doi.org/10.1007/s00406-019-01031-y

Mail, P. D. (2002). The case for expanding educational and community-based programs that serve lesbian, gay, bisexual, and transgender populations. *Clinical Research and Regulatory Affairs, 19*(2–3), 223–273. https://doi.org/10.1081/CRP-120013249

Matejkowski, J., Caplan, J. M., & Wiesel Cullen, S. (2010). The impact of severe mental illness on parole decisions: Social integration within a prison setting. *Criminal Justice and Behavior, 37*(9), 1005–1029. https://doi.org/10.1177/0093854810372898

Matejkowski, J., & Severson, M. E. (2020). Predictors of shared decision making with people who have a serious mental illness and who are under justice supervision in the community. *International Journal of Law and Psychiatry, 70*, Article 101568. https://doi.org/10.1016/j.ijlp.2020.101568

McAlpine, D. D., & Alang, S. M. (2021). Employment and economic outcomes of persons with mental illness and disability: The impact of the Great Recession in the United States. *Psychiatric Rehabilitation Journal, 44*(2), 132–141. https://doi.org/10.1037/prj0000458

Morales, E. (2013). Latino lesbian, gay, bisexual, and transgender immigrants in the United States. *Journal of LGBT Issues in Counseling, 7*(2), 172–184. https://doi.org/10.1080/15538605.2013.785467

Ng, H. H. (2016). Intersectionality and shared decision making in LGBTQ Health. *LGBT Health, 3*(5), 325–326. https://doi.org/10.1089/lgbt.2016.0115

Park, S. G., Derman, M., Dixon, L. B., Brown, C. H., Klingaman, E. A., Fang, L. J., Medoff, D. R., & Kreyenbuhl, J. (2014). Factors associated with shared decision-making preferences among veterans with serious mental illness. *Psychiatric Services*, *65*(12), 1409–1413. https://doi.org/10.1176/appi.ps.201400131

Peek, M. E., Lopez, F. Y., Williams, H. S., Xu, L. J., McNulty, M. C., Acree, M. E., & Schneider, J. A. (2016). Development of a conceptual framework for understanding shared decision making among African-American LGBT patients and their clinicians. *Journal of General Internal Medicine*, *31*(6), 677–687. https://doi.org/10.1007/s11606-016-3616-3

Peek, M. E., Odoms-Young, A., Quinn, M. T., Gorawara-Bhat, R., Wilson, S. C., & Chin, M. H. (2010). Racism in healthcare: Its relationship to shared decision-making and health disparities: A response to Bradby. *Social Science & Medicine*, *71*(1), 13–17. https://doi.org/10.1016/j.socscimed.2010.03.018

Pescosolido, B. A., Manago, B., & Monahan, J. (2019). Evolving public views on the likelihood of violence from people with mental illness: Stigma and its consequences. *Health Affairs*, *38*(10), 1735–1743. https://doi.org/10.1377/hlthaff.2019.00702

Rade, C. B., Desmarais, S. L., & Burnette, J. L. (2018). An integrative theoretical model of public support for ex-offender reentry. *International Journal of Offender Therapy and Comparative Criminology*, *62*(8), 2131–2152. https://doi.org/10.1177/0306624X17714110

Salyers, M. P., Matthias, M. S., Fukui, S., Holter, M. C., Collins, L., Rose, N., Thompson, J. B., Coffman, M. A., & Torrey, W. C. (2012). A coding system to measure elements of shared decision making during psychiatric visits. *Psychiatric Services*, *63*(8), 779–784. https://doi.org/10.1176/appi.ps.201100496

Say, R., Murtagh, M., & Thomson, R. (2006). Patients' preference for involvement in medical decision making: A narrative review. *Patient Education and Counseling*, *60*(2), 102–114. https://doi.org/10.1016/j.pec.2005.02.003

Schulman, K. A., Berlin, J. A., Harless, W., Kerner, J. F., Sistrunk, S., Gersh, B. J., Dubé, R., Taleghani, C. K., Burke, J. E., Williams, S., Eisenberg, J. M., Ayers, W., & Escarce, J. J. (1999). The effect of race and sex on physicians' recommendations for cardiac catheterization. *The New England Journal of Medicine*, *340*(8), 618–626. https://doi.org/10.1056/NEJM199902253400806

Seeleman, C., Suurmond, J., & Stronks, K. (2009). Cultural competence: A conceptual framework for teaching and learning. *Medical Education*, *43*(3), 229–237. https://doi.org/10.1111/j.1365-2923.2008.03269.x

Seo, J., Goodman, M. S., Politi, M., Blanchard, M., & Kaphingst, K. A. (2016). Effect of health literacy on decision-making preferences among medically underserved patients. *Medical Decision Making*, *36*(4), 550–556. https://doi.org/10.1177/0272989X16632197

Shen, N., Sequeira, L., Silver, M. P., Carter-Langford, A., Strauss, J., & Wiljer, D. (2019). Patient privacy perspectives on health information exchange in a mental health context: Qualitative study. *JMIR Mental Health*, *6*(11), Article e13306. https://doi.org/10.2196/13306

Toapanta, N., Salas-Gama, K., Pantoja, P. E., & Soler, M. J. (2023). The role of low health literacy in shared treatment decision-making in patients with kidney failure. *Clinical Kidney Journal*, *16*(Suppl. 1), i4–i11. https://doi.org/10.1093/ckj/sfad061

van Ryn, M., & Burke, J. (2000). The effect of patient race and socio-economic status on physicians' perceptions of patients. *Social Science & Medicine*, *50*(6), 813–828. https://doi.org/10.1016/S0277-9536(99)00338-X

Viruell-Fuentes, E. A., Miranda, P. Y., & Abdulrahim, S. (2012). More than culture: Structural racism, intersectionality theory, and immigrant health. *Social Science & Medicine, 75*(12), 2099–2106. https://doi.org/10.1016/j.socscimed.2011.12.037

Wright-Berryman, J. L., & Kim, H.-W. (2016). Physical health decision-making autonomy preferences for adults with severe mental illness in integrated care. *Journal of Social Service Research, 42*(3), 281–294. https://doi.org/10.1080/01488376.2015.1093580

4

YOUTH AND YOUNG ADULT SHARED DECISION MAKING

VANESSA V. KLODNICK, BRIANNE LaPELUSA,
REBECCA P. JOHNSON, ABBY MAYHUE, AND
DEBORAH A. COHEN

Transition-age youth (TAY) are an important high-risk subgroup of individuals with serious mental illness. Between the ages of 16 and 25, these TAY experience a period of rapid developmental change. This period of new responsibilities and roles is when serious mental health conditions (SMHCs) typically develop (Martel & Fuchs, 2017). SMHCs include serious emotional disturbance diagnoses (e.g., attention-deficit/hyperactivity disorder, conduct disorder) and serious mental illness diagnoses (e.g., bipolar, major depressive, and schizophrenia spectrum disorders; Centers for Medicare & Medicaid Services, 2019).

Compared with children and with middle-aged and older adults, TAY have the highest rates of SMHCs and the lowest rates of mental health service engagement (Substance Abuse and Mental Health Services Administration [SAMHSA], 2023). Successful, sustained transitions from child to adult service systems (typically occurring at age 18 in most states) are rare because child and adult mental health systems have different eligibility requirements, services, and expectations of an individual's responsibility for service engagement (Broad et al., 2017; Cleverley et al., 2020; Cohen et al., 2020; Cohen, Londoño, et al., 2023; Paul et al., 2015; Singh & Tuomainen, 2015). In child

https://doi.org/10.1037/0000478-004
Shared Decision Making and Serious Mental Illness, P. W. Corrigan (Editor)

services, families support the engagement of the young person, whereas in adult services, TAY are expected to support their own engagement (Walker, 2018). Neither child nor adult mental health services are designed for the developmental needs of TAY (Khetarpal et al., 2022). Young people can feel misunderstood and disrespected by mental health providers who focus more on treating symptom-related distress as opposed to focusing on what matters to young people: independent living, relationships, school, and work (Cohen, Londoño, et al., 2023; Klodnick et al., 2021; Klodnick, Johnson, et al., 2024; McCormick et al., 2023). The integration of shared decision making (SDM) philosophy and practice in community mental health services is promising for increasing TAY service engagement and improving outcomes.

As described throughout the book, SDM is a process in which mental health care providers and users collaborate and share knowledge to come to decisions about service plans. Making decisions about care based on mutually shared ideas is generally considered favorable because the outcome will be the product of shared principles and perspectives. SDM has been found to improve service satisfaction and attitudes toward recovery among adults with SMHC diagnoses in community mental health services (Aoki et al., 2022; Thomas et al., 2021). SDM is particularly promising for young people with SMHC diagnoses who may feel misunderstood and disrespected and may distrust mental health service providers. Although SDM concepts are generally valued in TAY mental health care, research describing and evaluating TAY SDM strategies has remained relatively scarce (Langer & Jensen-Doss, 2018). There is widespread support, though, for using SDM strategies to provide high-quality, resilience-based, recovery-oriented TAY mental health care (Center for Mental Health Services [CMHS], 2018; Heinssen et al., 2014; Mueser et al., 2015; Orygen, 2016; Sage, 2019).

In this chapter, we first describe the uniqueness of the transition-to-adulthood developmental phase for individuals with SMHC diagnoses that should be considered in SDM approaches. Then, we detail SDM approaches with young people who have received SMHC diagnoses, as documented in recent research. We end with policy, program, and practice design recommendations on how to best integrate SDM effectively into community mental health services for young people with SMHC diagnoses.

TRANSITION TO ADULTHOOD

The transition to adulthood (Martel, 2021) is a unique time in human development characterized by increasing levels of independence, instability, identity exploration, decision making, and self-focus (Aquilino, 2006; Arnett, 2023).

Multiple major shifts occur simultaneously related to role functioning and expectations, relationships, living arrangements, and vocational engagement (Aquilino, 2006; Arnett & Tanner, 2006; Lapsley & Edgerton, 2002). This time can be exciting, but it also can be stressful. Some researchers have described this developmental period as a lengthening of Erik Erikson's (1963) psychosocial adolescence stage (ages 12 to 18; see also Hochberg & Konner, 2020, and Stetka, 2017), whereas others have made the case that this developmental time has distinctly unique features and is better understood as emerging adulthood (ages 18 to 30; American Psychiatric Association, 2024; Arnett, 2000, 2023; Mitchell et al., 2021; see Figure 4.1). To better understand SDM practice with young people and associated challenges, one must consider both Erikson and Arnett's theories about transition-to-adulthood development.

Adolescence and Young Adulthood

Erikson (1963) described adolescence as a stage occurring between ages 12 and 18 that is rooted in exploration of independence and a development of a sense of self. The primary psychosocial conflict is *identity versus role confusion*, and the major question facing adolescents is, "Who am I?" Identity involves experiences, relationships, beliefs, values, and memories that make up a person's subjective sense of self. During adolescence, individuals try out different identities to figure out where they fit in society; being denied the opportunity to try out different identities can result in role confusion—for example, being unsure of who they are and where they fit; drifting to and from jobs, relationships, living situations, and commitments and feeling disappointed and confused about their place in life. A key experience during late adolescence is separation-individuation from family and caregivers. There is a redefining of the relationship between an individual and their family members as is evidenced when the individual reduces their dependency on family or caregivers to navigate society. Separation-individuation

FIGURE 4.1. Varying Age Group Definitions Based on Transition-to-Adulthood Theories

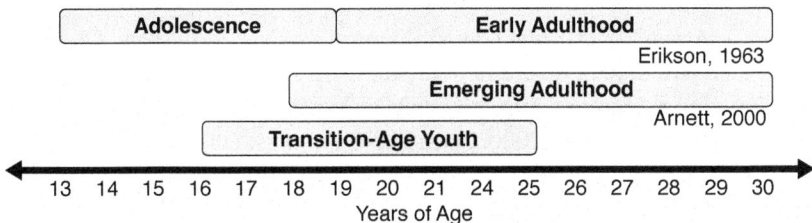

is achieved through a process of building independence and autonomy, developing goals and planning, and acquiring values and ethics. Adolescents become increasingly self-determined in the separation-individuation process.

Erikson (1963) defined *self-determination* in a variety of ways, but simply put, it is the idea that an individual determines their actions. Adolescents increasingly take on responsibility for their actions and decisions as they become young adults. In the United States and other capitalist societies rooted in individualism (as opposed to collectivism), adolescents develop responsibility for self as they try out different identities, friend groups, romantic partners, career paths, and living situations. This can be tricky because trying out different identities involves a certain amount of risk-taking that can make adults uncomfortable. However, it is an exercise important to moving into Erikson's young adulthood stage (between ages 19 and 40), when individuals face the major conflict of intimacy versus isolation in their navigation and development of strong close relationships with others (e.g., romantic partners, friends, colleagues). To make decisions about personal relationships, career paths, living situations, and community involvement an individual needs a certain level of self-understanding.

The transition to adulthood is a tricky life stage to navigate because this time is essentially a self-experiment through which one explores different situations, contexts, relationships, and communities to see how each feels. This self-exploratory period allows for the development of self-awareness so that the individual can make better life decisions to do things, choose environments, socialize, and love people in ways that bring joy, contentment, pride, and excitement. This process of self-exploration can be challenging, especially today, when young people face more life possibilities than ever before. Many have made the case that being an adolescent and young adult today is different than it was when Erikson published and refined his human development theory in the 1950s and 1960s and that this developmental phase starts later (Furlong, 2009; Haidt, 2024; Rubin et al., 2024; Twenge, 2017, 2023; Twenge et al., 2012).

Emerging Adulthood and Transition-Aged Youth

Jeffery J. Arnett (2000) first coined the term *emerging adulthood* based on more than a decade of qualitative research with TAY. He described this new developmental phase as different than Eriksons's adolescence and young adulthood stages (Arnett, 2000; Hochberg & Konner, 2020). Emerging adulthood typically occurs between ages 18 and 29 in industrialized countries and includes five core experiential elements (see Table 4.1).

TABLE 4.1. Five Core Developmental Experiences in Emerging Adulthood

Core developmental experience	Description
Identity exploration	Deep focus on developing who one is in society through exploration and experimentation
Age of possibility	Dramatic changes in identity and multiple life domains unlike any other time in the lifespan
Instability	Immense instability across all life domains (e.g., work, school, living situation, relationships, community engagement) compared with any other age group
Self-focus	Time in life with the fewest role obligations, caregiver/institutional monitoring, and commitments (emotional, financial)
Feelings in between	Not feeling like a child or an adult

Note. Data from Arnett (2000).

Arnett's (2000) theory of emerging adulthood is helpful for understanding young person logic and behavior. Emerging adulthood is defined by the feeling that one is in between childhood and adulthood—not fully identifying as adults responsible for meeting their own needs or the needs of others or identifying as children fully dependent on others (Arnett, 2000, 2023). During emerging adulthood, people experience new agency and self-focus in identity exploration through decision making and exploration of life's options. Physical, psychological, and emotional instability are core components of emerging adulthood (Arnett et al., 2014). Many emerging adults are not subject to the high levels of caregiver monitoring and oversight that they experienced during childhood, nor are they held to social expectations and responsibilities that they will face as adults, including to spouses, children, and community (Arnett, 2000, 2023). With privilege and resources, some young people have increasing time and access to explore and try out a multitude of identities and communities well into their late twenties.

Some feel an immense amount of pressure to figure it out while they are navigating change and instability during emerging adulthood. Individuals are no longer categorized as emerging adults once they take responsibility for themselves, make independent decisions, and become financially independent—typically around age 30 (Arnett, 2000, 2023). Young people must balance this newfound sense of responsibility with a deep desire to have fun and enjoy life during emerging adulthood before adult responsibility catches up with them. The social pressures of success, comparison, and self-image are accentuated by social media, which is evident in trends, such as the

30 before 30 Bucket List in which users compile a list of goals, fun experiences, and activities to complete before their 30th birthday (Afshar, 2025)—as if fun is destined to end at this age.

Resource access and social determinants of health—for example, socioeconomic standing, race or ethnicity, location or living situation, and disability (Centers for Disease Control and Prevention, n.d.)—affect the ability to explore and discover oneself in this way. In comparison with peers having fewer social barriers, young people who have less access to resources within their communities experience increased marginalization, stressors, and adult responsibilities and have less time or opportunities for self-exploration. Arnett's (2000) theory has been critiqued as being rooted in privilege and not being applicable to minority and marginalized youths and young adults (Bounds & Posey, 2022). In the United States in families with middle to high incomes, TAY tend to spend longer figuring out who they are as they change majors in college, change jobs, change relationships with peers, and change living situations well into their late twenties (Wood et al., 2018).

Many TAY, though, do not have the privilege of this lengthy self-exploration phase because of disadvantage, marginalization, and vulnerability (Sapiro & Ward, 2020); this group includes young people with SMHC diagnoses who tend to experience both delayed and accelerated transitions into adulthood depending on their unique circumstances. For example, TAY aging out of foster care tend to experience an immediate adulthood when they emancipate at age 18 or 21 depending on their state's policies (Munson et al., 2013). These vulnerable young adults often desire to live alone after years of living in heavily monitored group home settings to show that they can be independent because independence is what the child welfare system (e.g., judges, case workers) and treatment settings (e.g., therapists, psychiatrists) have emphasized as their emancipation goal (Klodnick & Samuels, 2020). Most young adults in the United States do not live alone at the age of 18 or 21. Navigating life independently is difficult financially and emotionally for these young people, who are more likely to face homelessness, psychiatric hospitalization, justice system involvement, trauma, and abuse in the year after aging out of care (Klodnick et al., 2021; Klodnick, Johnson, et al., 2024).

Overall, TAY with SMHCs have an increased risk for high school expulsion and dropout (or pushout), delayed high school completion, failure to enroll in or complete postsecondary education, unemployment and underemployment, comorbid substance use disorders, unplanned pregnancy and parenting, and justice involvement (Burke et al., 2023; Drake et al., 2013; Wagner & Newman, 2012). These experiences can limit possibilities in their careers, living situations, and relationships and can disrupt critical psychosocial developmental experiences. For example, they may miss out on meaningful extracurricular activities and part-time employment because their caregivers place higher priority on completing high school coursework that they may be behind on because of a psychiatric hospitalization or intensive outpatient treatment program. And many young people with SMHCs feel pressure from family members to apply for and continue using supplemental security income (SSI), a federal cash benefit available to individuals with disabilities that interferes with employment (Campbell et al., 2010). TAY with SMHC diagnoses are a growing group of SSI beneficiaries (Fraker et al., 2011). Families and young people can benefit from these monthly cash benefits that offset independent living expenses (Social Security Administration [SSA], n.d.). The problem is that young people tend to be in low-paying entry-level jobs with inconsistent hours (e.g., retail, fast food). In 2024, beneficiaries of SSI received $943 a month; making more than $943 from employment resulted in a reduction or loss of SSI benefits (i.e., by subtracting part of an individual's income from their disability check; Linebaugh & Chaikin, 2024). Young adults and their caregivers fear SSI benefit loss, which can thwart their engagement in competitive employment (SSA, n.d.).

TAY with SMHCs distinctly experience the "in-betweenness" that is common in emerging adulthood when interacting with child and adult mental health service providers. The child mental health system actively involves caregivers and may prioritize caregiver perspectives (Bjønness et al., 2022; Schnyder et al., 2020), which leaves young people feeling unheard and disrespected (McCormick et al., 2023). The adult mental health system, on the other hand, rarely involves family members and expects individuals to take full responsibility for their own care (Mulvale et al., 2019), which can feel confusing and frustrating (Cohen, Londoño, et al., 2023). Most young people with SMHC diagnoses live with family members and rely on family as they take on more personal responsibility during their transition to adulthood (Klodnick et al., 2021). One of the most challenging tasks young people with SMHCs face is navigating evolving formal (e.g., mental health professionals) and informal (e.g., caregivers, friends) relationships and social settings (M. Davis et al., 2011; Klodnick et al., 2021; Klodnick, Johnson, et al., 2024). Navigating evolving social and vocational roles and expectations is challenging for all TAY. However, TAY with SMHCs additionally face stigma, ableism, and social exclusion within their social network (Blajeski et al., 2022).

BETTER UNDERSTANDING AND EMBRACING TAY DEVELOPMENT

TAY with SMHC diagnoses who do not feel like they fit in either child or adult service systems is a testament to just how unattuned mental health service systems and providers can be with transition-to-adulthood development. Qualitative research with young people with SMHC diagnoses and intersecting disadvantage, marginalization, and vulnerability (Cohen, Londoño, et al., 2023; Klodnick et al., 2021; Klodnick, Johnson, et al., 2024; McCormick et al., 2023) has illuminated this misattunement. See Exhibit 4.1 for select quotes from young people navigating mental health services during their transition to adulthood. These studies sought to understand how and why young people engage and disengage in mental health services, especially when making the transition from child to adult service systems. Findings have suggested that young people overwhelmingly want mental health care but that their negative interactions with mental health providers and lack of access to desired services (e.g., therapy, employment, peer support) led most to disengage. Taking these current perspectives into consideration is important for

EXHIBIT 4.1. Transition-Age Youth Quotes Describing Young Adults' Mental Health Services

- "I never really felt like I was getting help. They [school counselors] would just tell my mom stuff. Someone told my mom that I had sociopathic tendencies and stuff, but they never tried to work with me on these issues that they said I had. They would just kind of talk about it with my mom." (McCormick et al., 2023, p. 532)

- "I did not appreciate the combative tone or the interrogative feeling of it [adult system intake]." (Cohen, Londoño, et al., 2023, p. 685)

- "It didn't feel like I was being asked questions to genuinely help connect me with services. It was more of like, 'Well why didn't you do this, this, and this, before you came here?'" (Cohen, Londoño, et al., 2023, p. 685)

- "I asked her [psychiatrist] questions afterwards, and she was like, 'Oh, I'm not comfortable sharing with you.' But I just got through sharing so much stuff about me with her!" (McCormick et al., 2023, p. 530)

- "I kind of didn't want to do [services] after the psychiatrist. Because he seemed rushed. . . . Not really paid attention to. . . . It didn't seem like he was listening to what I was getting at and saying." (Cohen, Londoño, et al., 2023, p. 683)

- "She [prescriber] tried to accuse me of lying one time when I tried to tell her how I felt about like how the pills were making me feel." (McCormick et al., 2023, p. 531)

- "Just the way [provider] was talking. The diagnoses that were coming up. I used Google. He's talking saying like, 'Well, this this this.' I'm like, 'Well, I'm here for one thing . . . seems like you're avoiding the one thing I keep telling you I'm here for.' He was just trying to give me stuff, diagnose me with stuff, instead of paying attention to what the problem is that I'm here for." (Cohen, Londoño, et al., 2023, p. 682) facilitating effective SDM practices with young people. See Figure 4.2, which illustrates the factors that cultivate trust and lead to service engagement.

For mental health systems and providers to become more developmentally attuned with TAY, they must shift to fully embrace both the notion of discovery and the concepts of recovery and resiliency. The concept of recovery drives many adult mental health programs in the United States (Ellison et al., 2018). *Recovery* is defined as "a process of change through which individuals improve their health and wellness, live self-directed lives, and strive to reach their full potential" (SAMHSA, n.d., para. 1). The concept of resiliency drives many child mental health programs in the United States (Ward, 2014). *Resiliency* is the capacity to cope with adversity and overcome threats to development (Davydov et al., 2010). The general notions of being self-directed, reaching one's full potential, and maintaining resiliency in the face of adversity all apply to young people with SMHC diagnoses. However, the word "recovery" connotes that people are getting something back or returning to some previous level or type of functioning. The notion of resiliency can, at times, be at odds with the risk-taking that is critical for young person's identity development. Self-discovery (and figuring out who one is in society) is a fundamental developmental experience that both Erikson (1963) and Arnett (2000, 2023) described as identity development in their transition-to-adulthood development theories.

TAY are typically developing self-knowledge for the first time as they experience developmentally appropriate seismic role shifts and new demands related to career, social network, family, and community while they simultaneously contend with their mental health symptoms. TAY are in various stages of integrating their mental health experiences into their still-forming identities. Young people profoundly feel the stigma of identifying as someone

FIGURE 4.2. Factors Leading to Transition-Age Youth Service Engagement and Disengagement

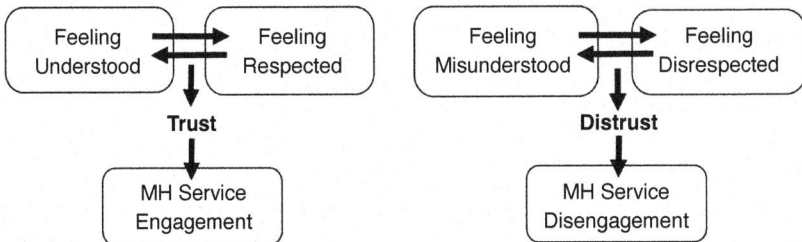

Note. MH = mental health.

with mental illness. Qualitative research has highlighted how traumatizing and dehumanizing SMHC symptom onset, diagnosis, and treatment can be in the wake of a first-episode psychosis, leading people to feel like they do not belong at work or in school settings (Blajeski et al., 2022; Dunkley et al., 2015; Fusar-Poli et al., 2022).

PROMISE OF SHARED DECISION MAKING

SDM is a promising philosophy and practice for boosting mental health service engagement and positive outcomes for young people. Youths especially do not appreciate being told what to do because they are increasingly taking responsibility for themselves as independent decision makers (Halpern-Felsher et al., 2016). SDM transfers power and expertise from the sole treatment provider (e.g., prescriber, therapist) to the individual with a SMHC diagnosis to ensure that the young person can make informed decisions about their care based on their personal preferences and goals.

SDM can be tricky with young people for several reasons. One is the involvement of caregivers or family either by law for youths younger than age 18 or by preference (or obligation) for those 18 or older. Well-intentioned adults want to protect young people from taking risks that may result in distress and hardship during an already stressful time in development. Adults and caregivers of young people with SMHCs specifically may be protective in ways that can limit SDM and inhibit the young person's growth and independence. For example, many caregivers may focus on mitigating risk by doing things for the young person, such as contacting mental health providers on their behalf, rather than doing things with or empowering them to practice skills on their own. However, it is through taking risks that young people learn about themselves and how to navigate society effectively. Reviewing and understanding treatment options may be difficult for young people depending on how the options are presented and described. Sometimes providers give young people and their self-identified family, caregivers, or supporters so much information that it is both cognitively and emotionally challenging for them to process let alone discuss and prioritize with key supportive adults.

Providers may focus more on clinical diagnoses and symptom psychoeducation than what young people care about most: navigating work, school, and relationships. Research has suggested that young people are more engaged when services and supports focus on the areas that are most relevant to their lives (Cohen, Londoño, et al., 2023; McCormick et al., 2023). Providers should shift to incorporate psychoeducation alongside this support when it is relevant to a young person's needs and priorities rather than make it a direct focus. Increasingly, efforts are underway to aggressively intervene on symptoms as early as possible after SMHC onset to prevent long-term disability-related struggles. As part of the SDM process with young people, providers and systems or institutions should embrace those youths' hesitations, questions, and pushback about the predominantly medical model approaches for treating SMHCs.

Power Dynamics in Shared Decision Making

Power dynamics among young people, families, providers, and systems affect SDM. In addition to the inherent power dynamics between client and provider, power differentials based on aspects of identity and experience further affect the ability for mutuality within decision making that is truly shared. Factors that include race, ethnicity, gender identity, sexual orientation, income level, education, and access to resources must be considered within the dynamics of SDM. Mutuality between providers and service users is an ongoing process based on mutual trust, authenticity, and respect within the relationship (LaPelusa et al., 2023; Lewis et al., 2016). A core value of peer support, mutuality describes the nonhierarchical approach to peer support relationships (Scott, 2011). All community mental health providers (with lived mental health experiences or not) can work toward establishing mutuality in their relationships with clients.

To increase mutuality for SDM with young people, all providers must gain awareness of their own implicit biases and how those biases show up within the power dynamics among themselves, young people, and systems or institutions. Providers must seek to understand the inherent effect of differences in identity, culture, and life experiences on power dynamics with young people. In addition, providers must recognize implicit biases related to race, ethnicity, gender, sexuality, disability, income, age, and other factors and examine how their life experiences and clinical training influence their approaches to SDM. For example, implicit biases and negative personal experiences related to substance use can create an instinctively parental dynamic between a provider and a young person who is curious about or is using substances. Further, it is crucial to fully consider the varying needs and circumstances of young people at every stage in decision making. Although existing research that defines transition age youth and emerging adulthood has been centered on middle- to upper class experiences (Côté, 2014; Hendry & Kloep, 2010; Wood et al., 2018), many young people enrolled in mental health services have a different hierarchy of needs, interests, vulnerabilities, and priorities for decision making. Providers and systems must understand and address power dynamics and differentials to authentically approach SDM with young people.

Barriers and Facilitators

Recent qualitative SDM research with young people and mental health providers has further illuminated the barriers and facilitators to integrating SDM with young people in mental health settings. Young people ($n = 10$; ages 16 to 18 years old) in inpatient mental health treatment in Norway reported that SDM prerequisites include accessible psychoeducation, mutual trust, and a strong working alliance between clients and therapists (Bjønness et al., 2020). Participants emphasized the importance of being involved in their own treatment from enrollment by cocreating treatment plans tailored to their individual needs and working together with their multidisciplinary team as an equal and respected partner. Being labeled with a diagnosis, forced into a standard treatment plan, and dominated by professional opinions (and rules) can elicit strong resistance in young people—like most people. A powerful experience rooted in communication, collaboration, and empowerment, SDM with young adults can be fostered—even in inpatient settings—when there is less emphasis on standardized assessment, diagnosis, and symptoms and an increased focus on building strong working alliances and individualizing treatment.

Another related qualitative study in Norway with 15 health care professionals in five different inpatient TAY mental health settings detailed the following five SDM facilitators: (a) involvement before admission, (b) sufficient time to feel safe, (c) individualized therapy, (d) access to meetings where decisions are made, and (e) changing professionals' attitudes and practices (Bjønness et al., 2020). These providers emphasized the importance of orientation and transition into an inpatient setting as well as inclusion of young people in decision-making spaces and personalized-care planning processes. SDM with TAY requires changes in agency culture and clinical assessment and treatment protocols that allow for more flexibility in individualized tailoring of mental health services that align with the young person's needs. Most importantly, perhaps, is how that study identified the critical need for mental health professionals to share the role of expert with young people (and their chosen social supports) as well as spend time explaining treatment approaches, listening to the young person's perspectives, answering their questions, and acting on that person's preferences.

Integrating these ideals is especially difficult in more medical model settings with long-established hierarchies of who is the expert and director of treatment (i.e., psychiatrists, psychologists, therapists) and who are the patients and recipients of treatment (i.e., TAY; Gravel et al., 2006). Akin to other evidence-based practice implementation efforts (e.g., trauma-informed care [Huo et al., 2023], supported employment [Bond & Mueser, 2022]), integrating SDM with young people requires organizational culture and practice shifts through leadership sponsorship, policy and program changes, and workforce development (Bond et al., 2023).

Shared Decision Making Processes: Perspectives of Clinicians, Transition-Age Youth

An Australian research team used qualitative methods with clinicians and young people at clinical high risk for psychosis to detail stages of mental health treatment decision making for TAY using the International Patient Decision Aid Standards and to identify challenges related to SDM with young people (Simmons et al., 2021). Unsurprisingly, clinicians and young people had different perspectives on SDM processes and related challenges. Clinicians identified three primary SDM stages in linear order: (a) the engagement phase, (b) the assessment and priorities for treatment phase, and (c) the initial and ongoing decision-making phase. During the engagement phase, young people decide whether they want to engage in treatment. The assessment and priorities for treatment phase is rooted in the individual's presenting symptoms and preferences for treatment and life goals. The initial and ongoing decision-making phase relies on collaboration, mutually sharing new information, and the monitoring of treatment responses from clients and families to inform treatment decisions. From the clinicians' perspective, challenges included getting on the same page while also sharing information about clinical high risk for psychosis that may be traumatic and stigmatizing, not over-clinicalizing the experiences of the young person, sharing language, and having discrepancies between what clinicians viewed as a treatment priority versus what the young person saw as a priority.

In contrast to clinicians, young people at clinical high risk for psychosis described SDM in a more relational and contextual way (Simmons et al., 2021). Young people emphasized the need to be involved, for their clinicians to be involved, and for clients themselves to be equipped with the knowledge and tools to take care of themselves and make independent decisions about their treatment. They described the importance of how information is shared and framed during SDM processes, how treatment engagement and goals inherently evolve for young people as they make progress on clinical goals and transition to adulthood, and how critical hope is for facilitating engagement in SDM processes. Young people were mixed in their perspectives of involving others (i.e., family members, nominated persons, peer support specialists) in SDM processes. Some reported family being heavily involved, and others did not have family involved (either physically or virtually) or reported that their involvement was unhelpful. Ultimately, young people emphasized that relationship building between providers and clients in addition to personal tailoring of care to their evolving unique needs and goals were necessary to promote effective SDM processes.

PROMOTING SHARED DECISION MAKING WITH TAY: PROMISING PRACTICES

Practice models and tools that support SDM among young people with SMHC diagnoses fall into the following categories: TAY advocacy or advisory boards, international systems change efforts, multidisciplinary mental health program design, near-age TAY and family peer support, and technology advances supporting TAY SDM. Table 4.2 presents practices, programs, and resources discussed next that promote SDM with TAY.

Transition-Age Youth Advocacy or Advisory Boards

TAY advisory boards center the expertise of young people to make shared decisions, advocate, and offer guidance within a program or organization. TAY-run advisory boards are emerging within youth programs to uplift youth voices; build community; and increase understanding around the needs, interests, and opinions of young adult participants in mental health programs (Guinaudie et al., 2020). Recent studies that involved the creation of TAY advisory committees have concluded that health professionals should engage with young people over an extended period to build meaningful relationships and recommended using incentives and offering training in skills, such as advocacy, to increase engagement of young people (Watson et al., 2023).

Several types of advisory boards exist. The following three offer slightly different approaches, purposes, and scope, and all are led by young people with lived (and living) mental health experiences.

1. Early Assessment and Support Alliance (EASA): This organization comprises young people from across Oregon who have graduated from EASA programs or who self-identify with psychosis. They convene monthly to

TABLE 4.2. Promising Practices for Promoting Shared Decision-Making With Transition-Age Youth

TAY approaches	Programs and resources for TAY SDM
Boards that involve and center young people in SDM processes within programs or agencies	• Early Assessment and Support Alliance Young Adult Leadership Council (https://easacommunity.org) • University of Massachusetts Transitions to Adulthood Center for Research Young Adult Advisory Board (https://www.umassmed.edu/TransitionsACR) • Thresholds' Youth & Young Adult Services advisory board (https://www.thresholds.org)

International systems change efforts	• United Kingdom
	   – i-THRIVE: https://implementingthrive.org
	   – MyMind: https://mymind.org.uk
	• Australia
	   – Headspace model: https://headspace.org.au

Coordinated specialty care for early psychosis	• Early Assessment and Support Alliance Connections (https://easaconnections.org) • OnTrackNY (https://ontrackny.org) • NAVIGATE team members' guide (https://navigateconsultants.org)

Transition to independence process model tools for teaching and supporting young people with SDM	• Transition to independence process model (https://www.starstrainingacademy.com):
	   – SODAS (problem solving and decision making)
	   – SCORA (conflict mediation method)

Near-age TAY and family peer support practices and approaches to SDM	• Achieve My Plan (https://achievemyplan.pdx.edu) • University of Massachusetts young adult peer mentoring (https://www.cbhknowledge.center) • OnTrackNY (https://ontrackny.org)
Policy and practice guidelines to integrate technology in SDM	Virtual Best Practice Guide for Youth & Young Adult Community Mental Health Providers (Johnson et al., 2022)

Note. TAY = transition-age youth; SDM = shared decision making.

shape the direction of EASA policies and practices across the state, providing nonstigmatizing information to inform SDM and creating peer support networks and communities of young people with lived experience with psychosis (Sage, 2019).

2. University of Massachusetts Transitions to Adulthood Center for Research Young Adult Advisory Board (YAB): The YAB comprises 18- to 30-year-olds from across the United States who self-identify with an SMHC. YAB members convene monthly to provide feedback on a variety of intervention research projects and related products (e.g., a peer-run podcast, meme development and dissemination) to promote work, school, and community participation among young people with SMHCs in the country (UMass Chan Medical School, n.d.).

3. Thresholds' Youth & Young Adult Services (YAYAS) advisory board: The board consists of young people with SMHCs currently enrolled in Thresholds' YAYAS programs in Illinois. The Thresholds YAYAS advisory board created a space that centers youth voices within the quality improvement activities of the YAYAS. Program staff (often peer support specialists) support TAY in participating in board activities and events and communicating information back to the programs. The board meets monthly, has several subcommittees working on a variety of initiatives, and meets with YAYAS leadership at least quarterly to provide feedback and ideas for YAYAS improvement (Thresholds, n.d.).

International Systems Change Efforts

In their youth/young adult mental health system redesign efforts, the United Kingdom and Australia have supported widespread adoption of SDM for young people with mental health needs. The United Kingdom designed and adopted a countrywide youth mental health systems change initiative called the i-THRIVE Framework (see https://implementingthrive.org) that includes SDM as a core practice principle (Wolpert et al., 2019). The i-THRIVE principles emphasize a common language understood by all—for example, children, young people and families codefine mental health needs with professionals through SDM. The initiative recognizes five different youth needs groups: those who are (a) thriving, (b) getting advice, (c) getting help, (d) getting more help, and (e) getting risk support. i-THRIVE has implemented initiatives to meet the needs of these five different groups—for example, developmentally attuned websites (e.g., MyMind website; see https://www.mymind.org.uk), school-based mental health teams, and early assessment and referral pathways to a community provider network (i-THRIVE, n.d.).

Australia's Orygen initiative is rooted in partnership with young people with lived (and living) mental health experience and aims to support the transition to adulthood for all youths in Australia through improved clinical care, research, education, advocacy, and policy and digital improvements (Orygen, n.d.) Orygen's clinical care efforts aim to be stigma free and support SDM with young adults and families. This initiative supports implementation of the *headspace model*, a community-based one-stop shop for young people needing support with their mental health, physical health (including sexual health), substance use, and vocational engagement (McGorry et al., 2019; Rickwood et al., 2019). Headspace uses SDM as a foundational practice (Rickwood et al., 2019) and has published several publicly available TAY SDM tools (Headspace National Youth Mental Health Foundation, 2012; Orygen, 2016).

Multidisciplinary Transition-Age Youth Mental Health Teams

Increasingly, team-based multidisciplinary care models are being recognized as best-practice for young people with SMHCs because of their constantly evolving needs and goals. In the United States, these teams comprise multiple specialty roles that embrace SDM philosophy and practices and typically include a clinically licensed therapist, prescriber, case manager, peer support specialist, family partner, and supported employment and education specialist (see Figure 4.3). Two leading multidisciplinary TAY-focused models in the United States include coordinated specialty care (CSC) for early psychosis (Heinssen et al., 2014) and the transition to independence process (TIP) model (Dresser et al., 2015).

Coordinated Specialty Care for Early Psychosis
CSC is a multidisciplinary, community- and team-based approach to early psychosis detection and intensive time-limited treatment (Read & Kohrt, 2022). CSC blends evidence-based practices and has a fidelity scale (Addington, 2021). Core principles of CSC for early psychosis include psychoeducation and SDM (Bello et al., 2017; Heinssen et al., 2014; Mueser et al., 2015). Studies that have investigated SDM experiences as related to CSC engagement have frequently concluded that SDM philosophies and practices make CSC experiences patient centered and individualized and thus are responsible for sustained young person and family engagement. The researchers explained how young people with early psychosis can choose their CSC services and specific providers within the CSC multidisciplinary team, and that doing so this leads to lengthier service participation (Hamilton et al., 2019; Zisman-Ilani et al., 2021).

FIGURE 4.3. Common Transition-Age Youth Team Roles

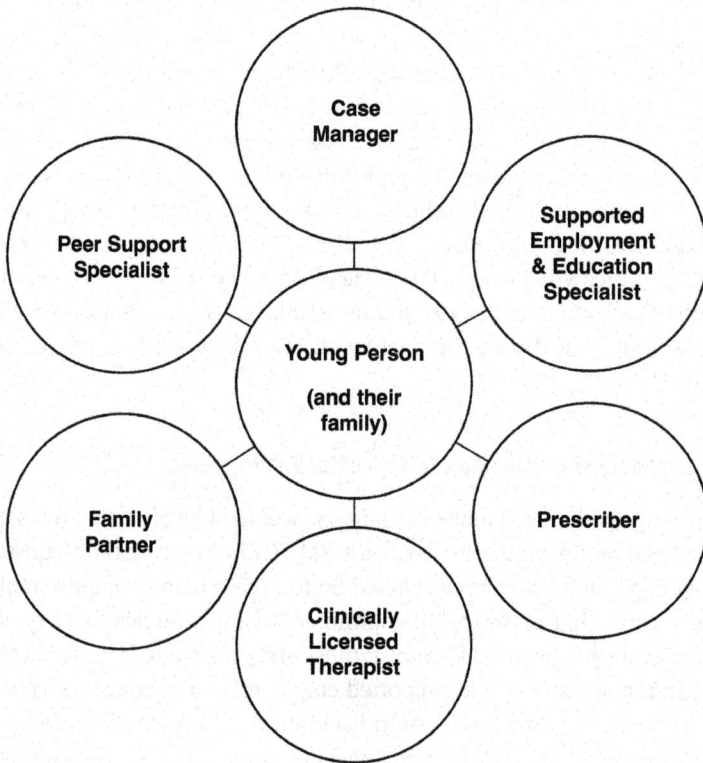

Peer support specialists use their own lived and living experiences with mental health and systems navigation to connect with young people and provide nonjudgmental support. Peer support offers a level of acceptance, understanding, and validation not found in many other professional relationships (Mead & McNeil, 2006). The peer support specialist is often cited as important in facilitating SDM processes, suggesting that who provides psychoeducation and how they provide it is important for understanding information, discussing information, making decisions, and acting on these decisions. One qualitative study examined barriers and facilitators to SDM among CSC participants ($n = 20$; Thomas et al., 2021). SDM barriers were related to information and knowledge factors (e.g., too much information can feel overwhelming, not enough information creates skepticism and limits perspectives), social/relational factors (e.g., lacking trust, strong working alliances with CSC team members), and internal patient factors (e.g., cognitive and communication challenges, low motivation; Thomas et al., 2020).

SDM facilitators were related to information and knowledge factors (e.g., having options and information to compare options), social/relational factors (e.g., stress relief when discussing options with trusted others, learning from observing and hearing about other CSC participants who are facing similar decisions); personal values (e.g., getting back to old self, making self and others proud), and time (e.g., having time to think about or talk through options; Thomas et al., 2020).

SDM guides for CSC are available. The Center for Practice Innovations that supports OnTrackNY CSC implementation across the United States has a set of videos to guide CSC providers in how to best use SDM with young people and families (Gingerich, 2020). The CSC model NAVIGATE has a CSC team member guide that includes specifics on collaborative treatment planning that is rooted in SDM best practices. The EASA early psychosis program in Oregon has a peer-driven website (EASA Connections; see https://easaconnections.org) with tools and resources to support informed decision making about CSC care (Raymaker et al., 2020), and a self-advocacy tool kit for TAY (EASA, n.d.). The National Association of State Mental Health Program Directors developed SDM recommendations for CSC teams to effectively transition young people when they complete CSC programming (Pollard & Hoge, 2022).

Transition to Independence Process Model
The TIP model is an application of the theory and practice of *positive youth development*, which is rooted in the idea that to engage and support healthy youth development, providers must foster young people's competence across social, cognitive, academic, and vocational domains; character; connections; confidence; and contributions (Arnett, 2023; Benson et al., 2006). TIP was designed to improve how child and adult service providers engage and effectively meet the unique developmental needs of 14- to 29-year-olds diagnosed with SMHCs. The TIP model practices support TAY goals across five transition domains: (a) personal effectiveness and well-being, (b) community life functioning, (c) educational opportunities, (d) employment and career, and (e) living situation. The TIP model is recognized as an evidence-informed practice (The California Evidence-Based Clearinghouse for Child Welfare, n.d.) and is currently implemented in more than half of the U.S. states.

The TIP model promotes SDM by increasing staff competency in teaching and by supporting young people in engaging in SDM as well as fostering problem-solving, decision-making skills, and learning through risk-taking and self-discovery. The TIP model uses a practice for social problem solving called *SODAS* (situation, options, disadvantages, advantages, and solution) to empower young people in making their own decisions, learning from them, and gaining new self-awareness (Skelton et al., 2016; Streetman et al., 2018). SODAS is a paradigm used to brainstorm different ways of social problem solving by exploring the options, advantages, and disadvantages within a situation (Pratt, 2022). The TIP model also uses *SCORA* (situation, concerns, options, review, agreement), a mediation practice to resolve conflict between young people and a third party (e.g., family member, roommate; Skelton et al., 2016; Streetman et al., 2018). The SCORA method uses a decision-making process for managing conflict by addressing concerns, exploring options, and reaching agreement with another person within a situation (Clark & Deschênes, 2021). The TIP model teaches young people and families to balance allowing for some risk so that young people can maximize learning while having their team as a safety net to both celebrate successes and make meaning of experiences perceived as unsuccessful (Dresser et al., 2015).

The TIP model also intentionally promotes and supports social network improvement and expansion to navigate the TIP transition domains more successfully. Developing and engaging in new friendships and romantic relationships are important developmental milestones during the transition to adulthood (Burt & Masten, 2009). Serious mental health symptom onset or exacerbation can drastically affect social functioning and relationships, including the ability and confidence to build new friendships and other social connections (Hodgekins, Birchwood, et al., 2015; Hodgekins, French, et al., 2015). The TIP model recognizes that who is involved (and how they are involved) in a TAY's services is dynamic, meaning that planning partners and necessary connections can and will change as a young person's goals and needs evolve across the transition to adulthood.

Near-Age Transition-Age Youth and Family Peer Support

Two new roles are increasingly being implemented on multidisciplinary teams to promote SDM among young people and family or caregivers: (a) the near-age youth/young adult and (b) the family partner. Youth/young adult peer support (YPS) is a unique new role that is increasingly common in TAY community mental health settings (Gopalan et al., 2017) and is important for promoting SDM practices and policies. Peer support is based on the idea that a person who has lived through adversity is uniquely positioned to connect with and promote positive outcomes for people experiencing similar challenges. *Near-age* typically means between 18 and 35, whereas *peer support* typically refers to using one's living or lived experience with a diagnosis of SMHC to support young people (typically between ages 14 and 26) with similar struggles (Halsall et al., 2022; Klodnick et al., 2015; Tawa et al., 2023). *Peer* is increasingly recognized to include shared characteristics and lived experiences beyond a mental health diagnosis and treatment, including but not limited to race, ethnicity, gender, sexual orientation, child welfare and justice system involvement, trauma, stigma, discrimination, and homelessness (Halsall et al., 2022; Ojeda et al., 2021; Walker et al., 2024). YPS values align strongly with SDM principles. YPS also values mutuality through cocreation, equity, the sharing and exploring of multiple perspectives, respect, community, and belonging (Tawa et al., 2023). YPS can take many forms, including engagement, emotional support, navigating and planning, advocacy, research, and education (de Beer et al., 2022).

To date, at least 18 U.S. states sponsor YPS training, professional development, or certification programs (Tawa et al., 2023). Many states have leveraged SAMHSA's Healthy Transitions initiative and system of care funding to introduce YPS roles into community health. These funding initiatives require youth voices and perspectives to systematically drive service design and implementation (SAMHSA, 2014). Part of the promise of the YPS role is that participants not only positively affect and support youth clients but also promote engagement and SDM practices in traditional clinical services (e.g., therapy, psychiatry) as well as use their youthful perspectives to inform program policies and practices (K. Davis et al., 2022; DuBrul et al., 2017; Tawa et al., 2023). Exhibit 4.2 presents a case example illustrating how Massachusetts designed and implemented a youth peer role across community mental health providers to support SDM practices.

The family partner role also is becoming increasingly common in child mental health systems, which serve young people up to age 21 in some states. The family partner uses their own lived experience of parenting a child experiencing mental health challenges to validate and support family members. Parents and caregivers of youths with mental health needs often experience barriers when attempting to access treatment, including structural barriers and lack of knowledge or understanding of mental health needs and the care-seeking process (Reardon et al., 2017). Family partners support families in effectively navigating treatment settings, schools, and individual education plans. Family partners teach self-advocacy skills and how to identify and access needed community resources and supports. Many U.S. states now have certified training programs for family partners.

Family partners can be helpful to the team SDM process because they support family members and represent the family perspective in team meetings. However, young people may not want to include a family partner in their treatment or decision-making processes for many reasons, including

EXHIBIT 4.2. Case Example: Youth Peer Support Implementation in Massachusetts

Initially funded through a Substance Abuse and Mental Health Services Administration system of care cooperative agreement from 2013 to 2017, the Massachusetts Department of Mental Health (MA DMH) engaged in a multiyear youth/young adult peer support implementation and role development process in its child mental health system. Young adult peer mentors (YAPMs) were initially hired and trained in 10 sites to serve 14- to 20-year-olds with mental health conditions who were enrolled in services at MA DMH and Mass Health (i.e., state Medicaid) behavioral health programs. YAPMs were paid employees who typically were between 21 and 30 years old, had personal lived mental health experiences, and supported young people by using these core elements: building relationships and collaboration; practicing cultural responsiveness; supporting young adult vision and goals; promoting self-care; role modeling; and (e) demonstrating safe, ethical, and professional behavior.

The YAPMs' practice profiles, 3-day training content, and organizational self-assessment tool are publicly available on the Massachusetts Children's Behavioral Health Knowledge Center's website (see https://www.cbhknowledge.center/). Today, more than 85 YAPMs are employed across a variety of settings (e.g., inpatient, residential, outpatient, access centers; Klodnick et al., 2023). These roles promote shared decision making (SDM) principles and practices across Massachusetts by ensuring young people's perspectives are heard and acted on in treatment planning meetings and while engaging in treatment. YAPMs meet monthly to support each other, brainstorm solutions, and identify challenges collectively experienced to be shared with MA DMH. This is an example of how a U.S. state is effectively embedding SDM with transition-age youth at systems and practice levels in community mental health.

Note. Case examples in this book are hypothetical.

a preference for autonomy (i.e., a desire to demonstrate independence in decision making) or privacy (e.g., for reasons ranging from annoyance to family dynamics that are overbearing and dysfunctional). Respecting a young person's boundaries with family involvement is crucial to establishing trust for SDM, especially for older youth and young adults. It is crucial that family partners explore their own parental or familial biases and maintain boundaries that align with the individual SDM preferences of clients and teams.

Awareness is increasing about the unique tensions between peer support (especially near-age peer support) and family partner roles in work with young people and families. Philosophical differences, though, exist regarding who sets priorities and who makes decisions in child and adult mental health care. Child systems actively involve family; adult systems typically do not (Cohen, Londoño, et al., 2023). More recently established (and growing) TAY systems are somewhere in between. The commonly implemented children's mental health approach Wraparound, for instance, is described as "Family Driven, Youth Guided" (Bruns et al., 2010, p. 2), whereas the adapted version of Wraparound for adolescents and young adults is called Achieve My Plan and is described as "Youth Driven, Family Guided" (Walker et al., 2012, p. 190).

This is an important distinction for the individual responsibility and participation of both young people and family caregivers in a youth's treatment. Some states have begun introducing both a near-age young adult peer support specialist role and a family peer support specialist role in TAY multidisciplinary teams and integrated mental health clinics (Cohen, Klodnick, et al., 2023).

In theory, this sounds ideal for SDM practice because participation by both young people and their families in mental health treatment is important for positive outcomes (Koroloff & Friesen, 2019; McGorry et al., 2022). However, in practice, it is complicated because these two roles have different perspectives, approaches, and priorities. For example, here's how a young person from Massachusetts described their early experience as a YPS specialist:

> It was hard in the beginning, especially because I feel like the [YPS specialist] role and the family partner role were a little bit oppositional. I'm here to advocate for the client and they're there to advocate for the parent—and a lot of the time the client and the parent are not on the same terms. But they're both roles where you get so invested because you come in with that 'I know what this feels like.' That was a big challenge in the beginning, really figuring out how to work effectively with the family partner. (Klodnick, Sapiro, et al., 2024, p. 534)

Technology Advances Supporting Transition-Age Youth Shared Decision Making

SDM tools that leverage technology are increasingly implemented and evaluated with young people with SMHC diagnoses to improve continuity of care and mental health outcomes. The smartphone is a critical tool for sharing information, involving young people and family in SDM processes and strengthening working alliances between clients and providers. Research has suggested that youths prefer texting over talking on the phone (Ehrenreich et al., 2020). COVID-19 led to widespread use of telehealth platforms and videoconferencing to deliver mental health care (McCormick et al., 2023). Videoconferencing allows for more people to be involved in mental health treatment–related SDM processes and for increased flexibility in providing support in real-time in the community in which young people are trying out new skills, taking risks, and gaining new self-insights. It is important for mental health providers to adopt virtual support and communication policies and practices to ensure that staff are using virtual tools in ethical ways based on client and family preferences. For mental health agency policy and practice guidelines to successfully integrate virtual tools to support SDM, review the *Virtual Best Practice Guide for Youth & Young Adult Community Mental Health Providers*, which was developed at Thresholds in Chicago during the COVID-19 pandemic (Johnson et al., 2022).

SDM smartphone applications and web portals allow care to be more person centered, treatment to be more tailored, and for clients and providers to collaborate more fully (Korsbek & Tønder, 2016; Vitger et al., 2019). A digital SDM intervention, Power Up for Parents, is promising for providing a safe space for parents or caregivers to ask questions, get needed information, and engage in meaningful discussion (Liverpool & Edbrooke-Childs, 2021). Power Up for Parents includes five elements: (a) decisions, (b) goals, (c) journey, (d) support, and (e) resources. An Australian study found that young people with depression who used a digital decision aid experienced high rates of treatment adherence, significantly reduced depression, and reported high satisfaction with the SDM tool (Simmons et al., 2017). Young people have shared that supplemental virtual support is not only helpful while in treatment but beyond discharge too (Montague et al., 2015). These studies mention struggles with implementing virtual SDM tools. To promote SDM through technology, the client's preferred mode of technology must be prioritized—and these tools must complement and supplement mental health care rather than completely replace evidence-based mental health services (Montague et al., 2015).

An Australian team piloted an online decision aid with 10 young people who were at clinical high risk for psychosis (Simmons et al., 2021). The online decision aid included guided psychoeducation around symptoms, risk factors, and treatment options presented on an accessible, easy-to-navigate website. The online decision aid described different treatment options; by clicking on each, users could learn more and access evidence-based information about the potential harms and benefits of each option and the likelihood of those outcomes. The aid also elicited personal preferences and values so that the person faced with the decision could work together with their treating clinician or team and any caregivers involved in their care. The decision aid was found to be acceptable and helpful in making treatment-related decisions: Of the participants, 8 of 10 chose at least one treatment approach, and at 6-week follow-up, 7 of 8 had continued with treatment. Treatments reported at follow-up included cognitive behavior therapy; schema therapy; cognitive analytical therapy; medications and vitamins; peer support; substance use counseling; and care coordination among school, family, and social services.

CONCLUSION

The transition to adulthood is a unique time in development with incredible shifts in an individual's personal responsibility, commitments, and independence—with major implications for SDM. Family members are systematically involved in child system mental health services but infrequently involved in adult community mental health services. During the transition to adulthood, young people with SMHCs age out of child system services, and legal decision-making authority (regarding mental health treatment) transfers from parents or caregivers to young adults as individuals. Best practices, including TAY-specific multidisciplinary team-based care promote SDM practices. Although there are some promising TAY SDM practices and interventions, more research is needed in the United States—especially in the emerging multidisciplinary and integrated programs. Research that explores young person and provider identity and demographic differentials (e.g., race or ethnicity, income level, education, resource access) is needed to further understand power dynamics and mutuality within SDM. Further, advisory board and near-age young adult peer support specialists benefit from informed and thoughtful support to successfully champion integration of SDM practices (Barba et al., 2022; Klodnick, 2019). As TAY programming continues to expand across the United States, there will be ample opportunities to better understand how different provider team member roles (with varying perspectives, approaches, and priorities) uniquely collaborate with young people, families, and others to support SDM goal attainment and recovery for young people.

REFERENCES

Addington, D. (2021). The first episode psychosis services fidelity scale 1.0: Review and update. *Schizophrenia Bulletin Open, 2*(1), sgab007. https://doi.org/10.1093/schizbullopen/sgab007

Afshar, M. F. (2025, January 8). Millennial woman asks what to do before turning 30—This was the response. *Newsweek.* https://www.newsweek.com/millennial-woman-asks-what-do-before-turning-30-2011631

American Psychiatric Association. (2024, January 16). *Not "just a teenage girl in her twenties": A new approach to human development.* https://www.psychiatry.org:443/news-room/apa-blogs/a-new-approach-emerging-adulthood

Aoki, Y., Yaju, Y., Utsumi, T., Sanyaolu, L., Storm, M., Takaesu, Y., Watanabe, K., Watanabe, N., Duncan, E., & Edwards, A. G. (2022). Shared decision-making interventions for people with mental health conditions. *Cochrane Database of Systematic Reviews, 2022*(11), Article CD007297. https://doi.org/10.1002/14651858.CD007297.pub3

Aquilino, W. S. (2006). Family relationships and support systems in emerging adulthood. In J. J. Arnett & J. L. Tanner (Eds.), *Emerging adults in America: Coming of age in the 21st century* (pp. 193–217). American Psychological Association. https://doi.org/10.1037/11381-008

Arnett, J. J. (2000). Emerging adulthood: A theory of development from the late teens through the twenties. *American Psychologist, 55*(5), 469–480. https://doi.org/10.1037/0003-066X.55.5.469

Arnett, J. J. (2023). *Emerging adulthood: The winding road from the late teens through the twenties* (3rd ed.). Oxford University Press.

Arnett, J. J., & Tanner, J. L. (Eds.). (2006). *Emerging adults in America: Coming of age in the 21st century.* American Psychological Association. https://doi.org/10.1037/11381-000

Arnett, J. J., Žukauskiene, R., & Sugimura, K. (2014). The new life state of emerging adulthood at ages 18–29 years: Implications for mental health. *The Lancet Psychiatry, 1*(7), 569–576. https://doi.org/10.1016/S2215-0366(14)00080-7

Barba, A., Klodnick, V. V., Munson, M. R., LaPelusa, B., & Johnson, R. P. (2022). *Bridging the gap peer kit for agencies of young adults in peer roles.* New York University Silver School of Social Work. https://socialwork.nyu.edu/content/dam/nyusilver/faculty-and-research/yyamh-g/btg-peer-kit-june-2022.pdf

Bello, I., Lee, R., Malinovsky, I., Watkins, L., Nossel, I., Smith, T., Ngo, H., Birnbaum, M., Marino, L., Sederer, L. I., Radigan, M., Gu, G., Essock, S., & Dixon, L. B. (2017). OnTrackNY: The development of a coordinated specialty care program for individuals experiencing early psychosis. *Psychiatric Services, 68*(4), 318–320. https://doi.org/10.1176/appi.ps.201600512

Benson, P. L., Scales, P. C., Hamilton, S. F., & Sesma, A., Jr. (2006). Positive youth development: Theory, research, and applications. In R. M. Lerner (Ed.), *Handbook of child psychology: Vol. 1. Theoretical models of human development* (6th ed., pp. 894–941). John Wiley & Sons.

Bjønness, S., Grønnestad, T., Johannessen, J. O., & Storm, M. (2022). Parents' perspectives on user participation and shared decision-making in adolescents' inpatient mental healthcare. *Health Expectations, 25*(3), 994–1003. https://doi.org/10.1111/hex.13443

Bjønness, S., Viksveen, P., Johannessen, J. O., & Storm, M. (2020). User participation and shared decision-making in adolescent mental healthcare: A qualitative study of healthcare professionals' perspectives. *Child and Adolescent Psychiatry and Mental Health, 14*(1), Article 2. https://doi.org/10.1186/s13034-020-0310-3

Blajeski, S. M., Klodnick, V. V., Caruso, N., & Sale, T. G. (2022). How early stigmatizing experiences, peer connections, and peer spaces influenced pathways to employment or education after a first-episode of psychosis. *Psychiatric Rehabilitation Journal, 45*(2), 144–152. https://doi.org/10.1037/prj0000502

Bond, G. R., Al-Abdulmunem, M., Marbacher, J., Christensen, T. N., Sveinsdottir, V., & Drake, R. E. (2023). A systematic review and meta-analysis of IPS supported employment for young adults with mental health conditions. *Administration and Policy in Mental Health, 50*(1), 160–172. https://doi.org/10.1007/s10488-022-01228-9

Bond, G. R., & Mueser, K. T. (2022). Supported employment. In W. E. Sowers, H. L. McQuistion, J. M. Ranz, J. M. Feldman, & P. S. Runnels (Eds.), *Textbook of community psychiatry: American Association for Community Psychiatry* (pp. 513–524). Springer International Publishing. https://doi.org/10.1007/978-3-031-10239-4_37

Bounds, D. T., & Posey, P. D. (2022). A resistance framework for racially minoritized youth behaviors during the transition to adulthood. *Journal of Research on Adolescence, 32*(3), 959–980. https://doi.org/10.1111/jora.12792

Broad, K. L., Sandhu, V. K., Sunderji, N., & Charach, A. (2017). Youth experiences of transition from child mental health services to adult mental health services: A qualitative thematic synthesis. *BMC Psychiatry, 17*(1), Article 380. https://doi.org/10.1186/s12888-017-1538-1

Bruns, E. J., Walker, J. S., Zabel, M., Matarese, M., Estep, K., Harburger, D., Mosby, M., & Pires, S. A. (2010). Intervening in the lives of youth with complex behavioral health challenges and their families: The role of the wraparound process. *American Journal of Community Psychology, 46*(3–4), 314–331. https://doi.org/10.1007/s10464-010-9346-5

Burke, C. W., Firmin, E. S., Lanni, S., Ducharme, P., DiSalvo, M., & Wilens, T. E. (2023). Substance use disorders and psychiatric illness among transitional age youth experiencing homelessness. *JAACAP Open, 1*(1), 3–11. https://doi.org/10.1016/j.jaacop.2023.01.001

Burt, K. B., & Masten, A. S. (2009). Development in the transition to adulthood: Vulnerabilities and opportunities. In J. E. Grant & M. N. Potenza (Eds.), *Young adult mental health* (pp. 5–18). Oxford University Press. https://doi.org/10.1093/med:psych/9780195332711.003.0001

The California Evidence-Based Clearinghouse for Child Welfare. (n.d.). Transition to independence process (TIP) model. Retrieved December 1, 2024, from https://www.cebc4cw.org/program/transition-to-independence-tip-model-2/

Campbell, K., Bond, G. R., Drake, R. E., McHugo, G. J., & Xie, H. (2010). Client predictors of employment outcomes in high-fidelity supported employment: A regression analysis. *Journal of Nervous and Mental Disease, 198*(8), 556–563. https://doi.org/10.1097/NMD.0b013e3181ea1e53

Center for Mental Health Services. (2018). *Assessing fidelity to coordinated specialty care for first episode psychosis.* National Association of State Mental Health Program Directors. https://coilink.org/20.500.12592/3fzg3b

Centers for Disease Control and Prevention. (n.d.). *Social determinants of health.* https://www.cdc.gov/about/priorities/why-is-addressing-sdoh-important.html

Centers for Medicare & Medicaid Services. (2019). *RE: Opportunities to design innovative service delivery systems for adults with a serious mental illness or children with serious emotional disturbance* (Publication No. SMD# 18–011). U. S. Department of Health & Human Services. https://www.medicaid.gov/federal-policy-guidance/downloads/smd18011.pdf

Clark, H. B., & Deschênes, N. (2021, August 1). *SCORA mediation method PPT 080121: Problem-solving/decision-making processes for transition-age youth & young adults.* https://docs.google.com/presentation/d/1LZz_klc52K7FfBahe1kcYgIW5wt34ygA

Cleverley, K., Lenters, L., & McCann, E. (2020). "Objectively terrifying": A qualitative study of youth's experiences of transitions out of child and adolescent mental health services at age 18. *BMC Psychiatry, 20,* Article 147. https://doi.org/10.1186/s12888-020-02516-0

Cohen, D. A., Klodnick, V. V., Kramer, M. D., Strakowski, S. M., & Baker, J. (2020). Predicting child-to-adult community mental health service continuation. *The Journal of Behavioral Health Services & Research, 47*(3), 331–345. https://doi.org/10.1007/s11414-020-09690-9

Cohen, D. A., Klodnick, V. V., Reznik, S. J., & Lopez, M. A. (2023). Expanding early psychosis care across a large and diverse state: Implementation lessons learned from administrative data and clinical team leads in Texas. *Administration and Policy in Mental Health, 50*(6), 861–875. https://doi.org/10.1007/s10488-023-01285-8

Cohen, D. A., Londoño, T., Klodnick, V. V., Emerson, K. R., & Stevens, L. (2023). "There wasn't any build up to it, it was just like, now you have to go over": Disengagement during the child to adult community mental health service transition. *Journal of Adolescent Research, 38*(4), 666–696. https://doi.org/10.1177/07435584221102914

Côté, J. E. (2014). The dangerous myth of emerging adulthood: An evidence-based critique of a flawed developmental theory. *Applied Developmental Science, 18*(4), 177–188. https://doi.org/10.1080/10888691.2014.954451

Davis, K., Chilla, S., & Do, N. (2022). *Youth and young adult peer support: Expanding community-driven mental health resources.* Well Being Trust. https://mhanational. org/wp-content/uploads/2024/12/Youth-and-Young-Adult-Peer-Support.pdf

Davis, M., Sabella, K., Smith, L. M., & Costa, A. (2011). *Becoming an adult: Challenges for those with mental health conditions.* https://repository.escholarship.umassmed. edu/entities/publication/04598bad-8259-43b5-8829-31797f8a7743

Davydov, D. M., Stewart, R., Ritchie, K., & Chaudieu, I. (2010). Resilience and mental health. *Clinical Psychology Review, 30*(5), 479–495. https://doi.org/10.1016/j.cpr. 2010.03.003

de Beer, C. R. M., Nooteboom, L. A., van Domburgh, L., de Vreugd, M., Schoones, J. W., & Vermeiren, R. R. J. M. (2022). A systematic review exploring youth peer support for young people with mental health problems. *European Child & Adolescent Psychiatry, 33*(8), 2471–2484. https://doi.org/10.1007/s00787-023-02163-2

Drake, R. E., Xie, H., Bond, G. R., McHugo, G. J., & Caton, C. L. M. (2013). Early psychosis and employment. *Schizophrenia Research, 146*(1–3), 111–117. https:// doi.org/10.1016/j.schres.2013.02.012

Dresser, K., Clark, H. B., & Deschênes, N. (2015). Implementation of a positive development, evidence-supported practice for emerging adults with serious mental health conditions: The transition to independence process (TIP) model. *The Journal of Behavioral Health Services & Research, 42*(2), 223–237. https://doi.org/10.1007/ s11414-014-9438-3

DuBrul, S. A., Deegan, P., Bello, I., Dean, E., Grossman, E., Chang, C., Watkins, L., Piscitelli, S., Lee, R., Ngo, H., Nossel, I., Vardin, A., Dixon, L., Dorr, M., Schwartz, E., & Stevens, T. (2017). *Peer specialist manual.* OnTrackNY. https://ontrackny.org/ Portals/1/Files/Resources/Peer%20Specialist%20Manual%20Final%202_17.17. pdf?ver=1-58SR66d_FI5NL5XawPRw%3d%3d

Dunkley, J. E., Bates, G. W., & Findlay, B. M. (2015). Understanding the trauma of first-episode psychosis. *Early Intervention in Psychiatry, 9*(3), 211–220. https:// doi.org/10.1111/eip.12103

Early Assessment and Support Alliance. (n.d.). *Self-advocacy toolkit.* https:// easacommunity.org/family-resource/self-advocacy-tool-3/

Ehrenreich, S. E., Beron, K. J., Burnell, K., Meter, D. J., & Underwood, M. K. (2020). How adolescents use text messaging through their high school years. *Journal of Research on Adolescence, 30*(2), 521–540. https://doi.org/10.1111/jora.12541

Ellison, M. L., Belanger, L. K., Niles, B. L., Evans, L. C., & Bauer, M. S. (2018). Explication and definition of mental health recovery: A systematic review. *Administration and Policy in Mental Health, 45*(1), 91–102. https://doi.org/10.1007/s10488-016-0767-9

Erikson, E. H. (Ed.). (1963). *Youth: Change and challenge.* Basic Books.

Fraker, T., Black, A., Broadus, J., Mamun, A., Manno, M., Martinez, J., McRoberts, R., Rangarajan, A., & Reed, D. (2011, April 5). *The Social Security Administration's Youth Transition Demonstration Project's interim report on the City University of New York's Project* (Mathematica Reference No. 06209.125). Mathematica Policy Research. https://doi.org/10.2139/ssrn.1849506

Furlong, A. (Ed.). (2009). *Handbook of youth and young adulthood: New perspectives and agendas.* Routledge. https://doi.org/10.4324/9780203881965

Fusar-Poli, P., Estradé, A., Stanghellini, G., Venables, J., Onwumere, J., Messas, G., Gilardi, L., Nelson, B., Patel, V., Bonoldi, I., Aragona, M., Cabrera, A., Rico, J., Hoque, A., Otaiku, J., Hunter, N., Tamelini, M. G., Maschião, L. F., Puchivailo, M. C., . . . Maj, M. (2022). The lived experience of psychosis: A bottom-up review co-written by experts by experience and academics. *World Psychiatry, 21*(2), 168–188. https://doi.org/10.1002/wps.20959

Gingerich, S. (2020, April 29). *NAVIGATE team members' guide.* NAVIGATE Consultants. https://navigateconsultants.org/2020manuals/team_guide_2020.pdf

Gopalan, G., Lee, S. J., Harris, R., Acri, M. C., & Munson, M. R. (2017). Utilization of peers in services for youth with emotional and behavioral challenges: A scoping review. *Journal of Adolescence, 55*(1), 88–115. https://doi.org/10.1016/j.adolescence.2016.12.011

Gravel, K., Légaré, F., & Graham, I. D. (2006). Barriers and facilitators to implementing shared decision-making in clinical practice: A systematic review of health professionals' perceptions. *Implementation Science, 1*(1), Article 16. https://doi.org/10.1186/1748-5908-1-16

Guinaudie, C., Mireault, C., Tan, J., Pelling, Y., Jalali, S., Malla, A., & Iyer, S. N. (2020). Shared decision making in a youth mental health service design and research project: Insights from the Pan-Canadian ACCESS Open Minds Network. *Patient, 13*(6), 653–666. https://doi.org/10.1007/s40271-020-00444-5

Haidt, J. (2024). *The anxious generation: How the great rewriting of childhood is causing an epidemic of mental illness.* Random House.

Halpern-Felsher, B., Baker, M., & Stitzel, S. (2016). Decision-making in adolescents and young adults. In M. A. Diefenbach, S. Miller-Halegoua, & D. J. Bowen (Eds.), *Handbook of health decision science* (pp. 157–167). Springer. https://doi.org/10.1007/978-1-4939-3486-7_12

Halsall, T., Daley, M., Hawke, L., Henderson, J., & Matheson, K. (2022). "You can kind of just feel the power behind what someone's saying": A participatory-realist evaluation of peer support for young people coping with complex mental health and substance use challenges. *BMC Health Services Research, 22*(1), Article 1358. https://doi.org/10.1186/s12913-022-08743-3

Hamilton, J. E., Srivastava, D., Womack, D., Brown, A., Schulz, B., Macakanja, A., Walker, A., Wu, M.-J., Williamson, M., & Cho, R. Y. (2019). Treatment retention among patients participating in coordinated specialty care for first-episode psychosis: A mixed-methods analysis. *Journal of Behavioral Health Services & Research, 46*(3), 415–433. https://doi.org/10.1007/s11414-018-9619-6

Headspace National Youth Mental Health Foundation. (2012). *Evidence summary: Shared decision making (SDM) for mental health—What is the evidence?* https://headspace.org.au/assets/download-cards/sdm-evidence-summary.pdf

Heinssen, R. K., Goldstein, A. B., & Azrin, S. T. (2014, April 14). *Evidence-based treatments for first episode psychosis: Components of coordinated specialty care* [Report]. RaISE. https://bhsoac.ca.gov/sites/default/files/nimh-white-paper-csc-for-fep_147096.pdf

Hendry, L. B., & Kloep, M. (2010). How universal is emerging adulthood? An empirical example. *Journal of Youth Studies, 13*(2), 169–179. https://doi.org/10.1080/13676260903295067

Hochberg, Z. E., & Konner, M. (2020). Emerging adulthood, a pre-adult life-history stage. *Frontiers in Endocrinology, 10,* Article 918. https://doi.org/10.3389/fendo. 2019.00918

Hodgekins, J., Birchwood, M., Christopher, R., Marshall, M., Coker, S., Everard, L., Lester, H., Jones, P., Amos, T., Singh, S., Sharma, V., Freemantle, N., & Fowler, D. (2015). Investigating trajectories of social recovery in individuals with first-episode psychosis: A latent class growth analysis. *The British Journal of Psychiatry, 207*(6), 536–543. https://doi.org/10.1192/bjp.bp.114.153486

Hodgekins, J., French, P., Birchwood, M., Mugford, M., Christopher, R., Marshall, M., Everard, L., Lester, H., Jones, P., Amos, T., Singh, S., Sharma, V., Morrison, A. P., & Fowler, D. (2015). Comparing time use in individuals at different stages of psychosis and a non-clinical comparison group. *Schizophrenia Research, 161*(2–3), 188–193. https://doi.org/10.1016/j.schres.2014.12.011

Huo, Y., Couzner, L., Windsor, T., Laver, K., Dissanayaka, N. N., & Cations, M. (2023). Barriers and enablers for the implementation of trauma-informed care in healthcare settings: A systematic review. *Implementation Science Communications, 4*(1), Article 49. https://doi.org/10.1186/s43058-023-00428-0

i-THRIVE. (n.d.). *Getting advice and signposting.* https://implementingthrive.org/about-us/the-needs-based-groupings/getting-advice-and-signposting/

Johnson, R. P., Schneider, A., LaPelusa, B., & Klodnick, V. V. (2022). *Virtual best-practice guide for youth & young adult community mental health providers* (Version 2). University of Texas at Austin. https://sites.utexas.edu/mental-health-institute/files/2024/09/Virtual-Best-Practices-Guide-Version-2-2022.pdf

Khetarpal, S. K., Auster, L. S., Miller, E., & Goldstein, T. R. (2022). Transition age youth mental health: Addressing the gap with telemedicine. *Child and Adolescent Psychiatry and Mental Health, 16*(1), Article 8. https://doi.org/10.1186/s13034-022-00444-3

Klodnick, V. V. (2019, July). *A guide to supervising and developing young adult peer mentors* (2nd ed.). Massachusetts Department of Mental Health. https://static1.squarespace.com/static/545cdfcce4b0a64725b9f65a/t/5d4afed3b302580001c43b9f/1565195999516/Supervision+Guide+for+YA+Peers_2nd+ed_July+2019_finalpdf.pdf

Klodnick, V. V., Gold, A., Pearlstein, M., Crowe, A., & Schneider, A. (2023). *Young adult peer mentors in Massachusetts: 2022 workforce details & needs.* Children's Behavioral Health Knowledge Center, Massachusetts Department Mental Health.

Klodnick, V. V., Johnson, R. P., Sapiro, B., Fagan, M. A., & Cohen, D. A. (2024). How young adults with serious mental health diagnoses navigate poverty post-emancipation: The complex roles of community mental health services & informal social support. *Community Mental Health Journal, 60*(4), 635–648. https://doi.org/10.1007/s10597-023-01188-w

Klodnick, V. V., Malina, C., Fagan, M. A., Johnson, R. P., Brenits, A., Zeidner, E., & Viruet, J. (2021). Meeting the developmental needs of young adults diagnosed with serious mental health challenges: The emerge model. *The Journal of Behavioral Health Services & Research, 48*(1), 77–92. https://doi.org/10.1007/s11414-020-09699-0

Klodnick, V. V., Sabella, K., Brenner, C. J., Krzos, I. M., Ellison, M. L., Kaiser, S. M., Davis, M., & Fagan, M. A. (2015). Perspectives of young emerging adults with serious mental health conditions on vocational peer mentors. *Journal of*

Emotional and Behavioral Disorders, *23*(4), 226–237. https://doi.org/10.1177/1063426614565052

Klodnick, V. V., & Samuels, G. M. (2020). Building home on a fault line: Aging out of child welfare with a serious mental health diagnosis. *Child & Family Social Work*, *25*(3), 704–713. https://doi.org/10.1016/j.childyouth.2013.03.003

Klodnick, V. V., Sapiro, B., Gold, A., Pearlstein, M., Crowe, A. N., Schneider, A., Johnson, R. P., LaPelusa, B., & Holland, H. (2024). Relational complexity of the near-age peer support provider role in youth & young adult community mental health settings. *The Journal of Behavioral Health Services & Research*, *51*(4), 545–560. https://doi.org/10.1007/s11414-024-09877-4

Koroloff, N., & Friesen, B. (2019, March 3–6). *Family roles in the transition of young adults with mental health conditions* [Conference session]. 32nd Annual Research & Policy Conference on Child, Adolescent, and Young Adult Behavioral Health, Tampa, FL, United States. https://www.cmhnetwork.org/wp-content/uploads/2019/04/S23B-KOROLOFF.pdf

Korsbek, L., & Tønder, E. S. (2016). Momentum: A smartphone application to support shared decision making for people using mental health services. *Psychiatric Rehabilitation Journal*, *39*(2), 167–172. https://doi.org/10.1037/prj0000173

Langer, D. A., & Jensen-Doss, A. (2018). Shared decision-making in youth mental health care: Using the evidence to plan treatments collaboratively. *Journal of Clinical Child & Adolescent Psychology*, *47*(5), 821–831. https://doi.org/10.1080/15374416.2016.1247358

LaPelusa, B., Klodnick, V., Reznik, S., & Johnson, R. (2023). *Peer approaches to substances for early psychosis programs (PAS-EPP): A toolkit for CSC peer providers.* University of Texas at Austin, The Texas Institute for Excellence in Mental Health.

Lapsley, D. K., & Edgerton, J. (2002). Separation-individuation, adult attachment style, and college adjustment. *Journal of Counseling and Development*, *80*(4), 484–492. https://doi.org/10.1002/j.1556-6678.2002.tb00215.x

Lewis, L., Tew, J., Ecclestone, K., & Spandler, H. (2016). *Mutuality, wellbeing and mental health recovery: Exploring the roles of creative arts adult community learning and participatory arts initiatives.* Education Observatory. https://educationobservatory.co.uk/wp-content/uploads/2018/05/CC-Full-Final.pdf

Linebaugh, M., & Chaikin, D. (2024, April 4). *How much can you work while receiving SSI disability benefits?* NOLO. https://www.nolo.com/legal-encyclopedia/how-much-can-you-work-while-receiving-ssi-disability-benefits.html

Liverpool, S., & Edbrooke-Childs, J. (2021). A caregiver digital intervention to support shared decision making in child and adolescent mental health services: Development process and stakeholder involvement analysis. *JMIR Formative Research*, *5*(6), Article e24896. https://doi.org/10.2196/24896

Martel, A. (2021). Transition-age youth: Who are they? What are their unique developmental needs? How can mental health practitioners support them? In V. Chan & J. Derenne (Eds.), *Transition-age youth mental health care: Bridging the gap between pediatric and adult psychiatric care* (pp. 3–42). Springer. https://doi.org/10.1007/978-3-030-62113-1_1

Martel, A., & Fuchs, D. C. (2017). Transitional age youth and mental illness—Influences on young adult outcomes. *Child and Adolescent Psychiatric Clinics of North America*, *26*(2), xiii–xvii. https://doi.org/10.1016/j.chc.2017.01.001

McCormick, K. A., Chatham, A., Klodnick, V. V., Schoenfeld, E. A., & Cohen, D. A. (2023). Mental health service experiences among transition-age youth: Interpersonal continuums that influence engagement in care. *Child and Adolescent Social Work Journal, 40*, 525–536. https://doi.org/10.1007/s10560-022-00890-0

McGorry, P., Trethowan, J., & Rickwood, D. (2019). Creating headspace for integrated youth mental health care. *World Psychiatry, 18*(2), 140–141. https://doi.org/10.1002/wps.20619

McGorry, P. D., Mei, C., Chanen, A., Hodges, C., Alvarez-Jimenez, M., & Killackey, E. (2022). Designing and scaling up integrated youth mental health care. *World Psychiatry, 21*(1), 61–76. https://doi.org/10.1002/wps.20938

Mead, S., & McNeil, C. (2006). Peer support: what makes it unique? *International Journal of Psychosocial Rehabilitation, 10*(2), 29–37.

Mitchell, L. L., Lodi-Smith, J., Baranski, E. N., & Whitbourne, S. K. (2021). Implications of identity resolution in emerging adulthood for intimacy, generativity, and integrity across the adult lifespan. *Psychology and Aging, 36*(5), 545–556. https://doi.org/10.1037/pag0000537

Montague, A. E., Varcin, K. J., Simmons, M. B., & Parker, A. G. (2015). Putting technology into youth mental health practice: Young people's perspectives. *Sage Open, 5*(2). https://doi.org/10.1177/2158244015581019

Mueser, K. T., Penn, D. L., Addington, J., Brunette, M. F., Gingerich, S., Glynn, S. M., Lynde, D. W., Gottlieb, J. D., Meyer-Kalos, P., McGurk, S. R., Cather, C., Saade, S., Robinson, D. G., Schooler, N. R., Rosenheck, R. A., & Kane, J. M. (2015). The NAVIGATE program for first-episode psychosis: Rationale, overview, and description of psychosocial components. *Psychiatric Services, 66*(7), 680–690. https://doi.org/10.1176/appi.ps.201400413

Mulvale, G. M., Nguyen, T. D., Miatello, A. M., Embrett, M. G., Wakefield, P. A., & Randall, G. E. (2019). Lost in transition or translation? Care philosophies and transitions between child and youth and adult mental health services: A systematic review. *Journal of Mental Health, 28*(4), 379–388. https://doi.org/10.3109/09638237.2015.1124389

Munson, M. R., Lee, B. R., Miller, D., Cole, A., & Nedelcu, C. (2013). Emerging adulthood among former system youth: The ideal versus the real. *Children and Youth Services Review, 35*(6), 923–929. https://doi.org/10.1016/j.childyouth.2013.03.003

Ojeda, V. D., Jones, N., Munson, M. R., Berliant, E., & Gilmer, T. P. (2021). Roles of peer specialists and use of mental health services among youth with serious mental illness. *Early Intervention in Psychiatry, 15*(4), 914–921. https://doi.org/10.1111/eip.13036

Orygen. (n.d.). *Orygen strategy 2022–2027.* https://www.orygen.org.au/getattachment/About/Strategic-plan/Orygen-Strategic-Plan-2022-2027-A4-web.pdf.aspx?lang=en-AU

Orygen. (2016). *Clinical practice in youth mental health: Shared decision making.* https://www.orygen.org.au/Training/Resources/General-resources/Clinical-practice-points/Shared-decision-making/Shared-decision-making

Paul, M., Street, C., Wheeler, N., & Singh, S. P. (2015). Transition to adult services for young people with mental health needs: A systematic review. *Clinical Child Psychology and Psychiatry, 20*(3), 436–457. https://doi.org/10.1177/1359104514526603

Pollard, J., & Hoge, M. (2022). *Transitioning clients from coordinated specialty care: A guide for clinicians.* National Association of State Mental Health Program Directors. https://www.ctearlypsychosisnetwork.org/uploads/1/3/4/8/134898305/guidance_document_transitions_csc_providers.pdf

Pratt, D. (2022). *Making the most informed choice: The SODAS problem-solving model.* PESI. https://www.pesi.com/blog/details/2048/making-the-most-informed-choice-the-sodas-problem-solving

Raymaker, D. M., Sale, T., Rija, M., Buekea, N., Caruso, N., Melton, R., Cohrs, N., Gould, V., Wall, C., & Scharer, M. (2020). Early assessment and support alliance connections: Community-based participatory research to develop a peer-based early psychosis web resource with young adults. *Progress in Community Health Partnerships: Research, Education, and Action, 14*(4), 471–480. https://doi.org/10.1353/cpr.2020.0052

Read, H., & Kohrt, B. A. (2022). The history of coordinated specialty care for early intervention in psychosis in the United States: A review of effectiveness, implementation, and fidelity. *Community Mental Health Journal, 58*(5), 835–846. https://doi.org/10.1007/s10597-021-00891-w

Reardon, T., Harvey, K., Baranowska, M., O'Brien, D., Smith, L., & Creswell, C. (2017). What do parents perceive are the barriers and facilitators to accessing psychological treatment for mental health problems in children and adolescents? A systematic review of qualitative and quantitative studies. *European Child & Adolescent Psychiatry, 26*(6), 623–647. https://doi.org/10.1007/s00787-016-0930-6

Rickwood, D., Paraskakis, M., Quin, D., Hobbs, N., Ryall, V., Trethowan, J., & McGorry, P. (2019). Australia's innovation in youth mental health care: The Headspace Centre model. *Early Intervention in Psychiatry, 13*(1), 159–166. https://doi.org/10.1111/eip.12740

Rubin, J. D., Chen, K., & Tung, A. (2024). Generation Z's challenges to financial independence: Adolescents' and early emerging adults' perspectives on their financial futures. *Journal of Adolescent Research.* Advance online publication. https://doi.org/10.1177/07435584241256572

Sage, M. G. (Ed.). (2019). *EASA participant manual.* EASA. https://easacommunity.org/wp-content/uploads/2023/09/EASA-Participant-Manual.pdf

Sapiro, B., & Ward, A. (2020). Marginalized youth, mental health, and connection with others: A review of the literature. *Child and Adolescent Social Work Journal, 37*, 343–357. https://doi.org/10.1007/s10560-019-00628-5

Schnyder, N., Lawrence, D., Panczak, R., Sawyer, M. G., Whiteford, H. A., Burgess, P. M., & Harris, M. G. (2020). Perceived need and barriers to adolescent mental health care: Agreement between adolescents and their parents. *Epidemiology and Psychiatric Sciences, 29*, Article e60. https://doi.org/10.1017/S2045796019000568

Scott, A. (2011). Authenticity work: Mutuality and boundaries in peer support. *Society and Mental Health, 1*(3), 173–184. https://doi.org/10.1177/2156869311431101

Simmons, M. B., Brushe, M., Elmes, A., Polari, A., Nelson, B., & Montague, A. (2021). Shared decision making with young people at ultra high risk of psychotic disorder. *Frontiers in Psychiatry, 12*, Article 683775. https://doi.org/10.3389/fpsyt.2021.683775

Simmons, M. B., Elmes, A., McKenzie, J. E., Trevena, L., & Hetrick, S. E. (2017). Right choice, right time: Evaluation of an online decision aid for youth depression. *Health Expectations, 20*(4), 714–723. https://doi.org/10.1111/hex.12510

Singh, S. P., & Tuomainen, H. (2015). Transition from child to adult mental health services: Needs, barriers, experiences and new models of care. *World Psychiatry*, *14*(3), 358–361. https://doi.org/10.1002/wps.20266

Skelton, E. A., Crosland, K. A., & Clark, H. B. (2016). Acquisition of a social problem-solving method by caregivers in the foster care system: Evaluation and implications. *Child & Family Behavior Therapy*, *38*(1), 32–46. https://doi.org/10.1080/07317107.2016.1135699

Social Security Administration. (n.d.). *Youth transition demonstration (YTD)*. https://www.ssa.gov/disabilityresearch/youth.htm

Stetka, B. (2017, September 19). Extended adolescence: When 25 is the new 18. *Scientific American*. https://www.scientificamerican.com/article/extended-adolescence-when-25-is-the-new-181/

Streetman, C., Crosland, K., & Clark, H. B. (2018). The acquisition and usage of the SODAS problem-solving method among adults at risk for homelessness. *Research on Social Work Practice*, *28*(8), 943–951. https://doi.org/10.1177/1049731516662318

Substance Abuse and Mental Health Services Administration. (n.d.). *Recovery and recovery support*. https://www.samhsa.gov/find-help/recovery

Substance Abuse and Mental Health Services Administration. (2014). *"Now is the Time" Healthy Transitions (HT): Improving Life Trajectories for Youth and Young Adults With, or at Risk for, Serious Mental Health Conditions* (Request for Applications No. SM-14-017). https://www.samhsa.gov/sites/default/files/grants/pdf/sm-14-017_0.pdf

Substance Abuse and Mental Health Services Administration. (2023). *Key substance use and mental health indicators in the United States: Results from the 2022 National Survey on Drug Use and Health* (HHS Publication No. PEP23-07-01-006, NSDUH Series H-58). https://www.cdc.gov/overdose-prevention/media/pdfs/2024/04/SAMHSA-Key-substance-use-and-mental-health-indicators-2022.pdf

Tawa, K., Kim, E., & Howdershelt, M. (2023, July). *Giving the young people what they want: A policy framework for youth peer support*. The Center for Law and Social Policy. https://www.clasp.org/wp-content/uploads/2023/07/2023.7.27_Youth-Peer-Support-Report.pdf

Thomas, E. C., Ben-David, S., Treichler, E., Roth, S., Dixon, L. B., Salzer, M., & Zisman-Ilani, Y. (2021). A systematic review of shared decision-making interventions for service users with serious mental illnesses: State of the science and future directions. *Psychiatric Services*, *72*(11), 1288–1300. https://doi.org/10.1176/appi.ps.202000429

Thomas, E. C., Snethen, G., & Salzer, M. S. (2020). Community participation factors and poor neurocognitive functioning among persons with schizophrenia. *American Journal of Orthopsychiatry*, *90*(1), 90–97. https://doi.org/10.1037/ort0000399

Thresholds. (n.d.). *Youth & young adult services*. https://www.thresholds.org/programs-services/youth-young-adult-services

Twenge, J. M. (2017). *iGen: Why today's super-connected kids are growing up less rebellious, more tolerant, less happy—And completely unprepared for adulthood—And what that means for the rest of us*. Atria Books.

Twenge, J. M. (2023). *Generations: The real differences between Gen Z, Millennials, Gen X, Boomers, and Silents—And what they mean for the future*. Atria Paperback.

Twenge, J. M., Campbell, W. K., & Freeman, E. C. (2012). Generational differences in young adults' life goals, concern for others, and civic orientation, 1966–2009. *Journal of Personality and Social Psychology, 102*(5), 1045–1062. https://doi.org/10.1037/a0027408

UMass Chan Medical School. (n.d.). *Transitions to Adulthood Center for Research (Transitions ACR): Young Adult Advisory Board (YAB).* https://www.umassmed.edu/TransitionsACR/about-us/youth-voice-and-participatory-action-research/YAB/

Vitger, T., Austin, S. F., Petersen, L., Tønder, E. S., Nordentoft, M., & Korsbek, L. (2019). The Momentum trial: The efficacy of using a smartphone application to promote patient activation and support shared decision making in people with a diagnosis of schizophrenia in outpatient treatment settings: A randomized controlled single-blind trial. *BMC Psychiatry, 19*(1), Article 185. https://doi.org/10.1186/s12888-019-2143-2

Wagner, M., & Newman, L. (2012). Longitudinal transition outcomes of youth with emotional disturbances. *Psychiatric Rehabilitation Journal, 35*(3), 199–208. https://doi.org/10.2975/35.3.2012.199.208

Walker, J. S. (2018). *A screeching halt: Family involvement when a youth with mental health needs turns 18: Commentary on state of the science from a family perspective.* Research and Training Center for Pathways to Positive Futures, Portland State University.

Walker, J. S., Klodnick, V. V., LaPelusa, B., Blajeski, S. M., Freedman, A. R., & Marble, S. (2024). A theory of change for one-on-one peer support for older adolescents and young adults. *Children and Youth Services Review, 157*, Article 107386. https://doi.org/10.1016/j.childyouth.2023.107386

Walker, J. S., Pullmann, M. D., Moser, C. L., & Burns, E. J. (2012). Does team-based planning "work" for adolescents? Findings from studies of wraparound. *Psychiatric Rehabilitation Journal, 35*(3), 189–198. https://doi.org/10.2975/35.3.2012.189.198

Ward, D. (2014). "Recovery": Does it fit for adolescent mental health? *Journal of Child & Adolescent Mental Health, 26*(1), 83–90. https://doi.org/10.2989/17280583.2013.877465

Watson, D., Mhlaba, M., Molelekeng, G., Chauke, T. A., Simao, S. C., Jenner, S., Ware, L. J., & Barker, M. (2023). How do we best engage young people in decision-making about their health? A scoping review of deliberative priority setting methods. *International Journal for Equity in Health, 22*(1), Article 17. https://doi.org/10.1186/s12939-022-01794-2

Wolpert, M., Harris, R., Hodges, S., Fuggle, P., James, R., Wiener, A., McKenna, C., Law, D., York, A., Jones, M., Fonagy, P., Fleming, I., & Munk, S. (2019). *THRIVE framework for system change.* CAMHS Press. https://implementingthrive.org/wp-content/uploads/2019/03/THRIVE-Framework-for-system-change-2019.pdf

Wood, D., Crapnell, T., Lau, L., Bennett, A., Lotstein, D., Ferris, M., & Kuo, A. (2018). Emerging adulthood as a critical stage in the life course. In N. Halfon, C. B. Forrest, R. M. Lerner, & E. M. Faustman (Eds.), *Handbook of life course health development* (pp. 123–143). Springer. https://doi.org/10.1007/978-3-319-47143-3_27

Zisman-Ilani, Y., Roth, R. M., & Mistler, L. A. (2021). Time to support extensive implementation of shared decision making in psychiatry. *JAMA Psychiatry, 78*(11), 1183–1184. https://doi.org/10.1001/jamapsychiatry.2021.2247

5 DECISION MAKING, RECOVERY, AND PEER SUPPORT

KARYN BOLDEN STOVALL AND LINDSAY SHEEHAN

This chapter focuses on the special role of peer support (both mutual mechanisms as well as formal peer services) in recovery and decision making. *Peer* is defined as a person with lived experience; for this book, this definition includes both the firsthand experience of mental illness and shared identities related to co-occurring disorders (e.g., substance use, human immunodeficiency virus, acquired immune deficiency syndrome) or to structural barriers and social disadvantage. Disclosure, the key part of being a peer, is unpacked in this chapter. We begin by exploring a brief history of peer support, the current state of shared decision making (SDM), and how SDM can fundamentally support those living with mental health conditions to grow and thrive.

HISTORY OF PEER SUPPORT

To begin, it is imperative to understand the history of peer support from both an international and a domestic perspective. The history of peer support within the behavioral health field is often traced to Jean-Baptiste Pussin in

https://doi.org/10.1037/0000478-005
Shared Decision Making and Serious Mental Illness, P. W. Corrigan (Editor)

18th century France. Pussin worked in the Bicêtre Hospital and hired patients who were in recovery to provide services to others living with similar conditions (Schuster et al., 2011). He was one of the first in the mental health field to work toward creating a treatment atmosphere that treated patients humanely. Moreover, he worked to improve the living conditions of hospitalized patients by reducing the usage of chains to confine patients and increasing their food rations.

Almost a century later in 1845, the Alleged Lunatics' Friend Society was created to advocate for patients to receive support for their mental health challenges (Van Tosh et al., 2000). Indeed, at the heart of much of the peer support implementation and changes over the years has been the fight for justice and equality. Few exemplify this fight better than Elizabeth Packard, who, in 1864, went to trial to defend herself after being committed by her husband to the Illinois Hospital for several years (Himelhoch & Shaffer, 1979). At that time, husbands could have their wives committed with little to no evidence of mental illness. After winning her trial and being released from the hospital, she spent the rest of her days advocating for the rights of women and those with mental illness.

In the 1900s, more progress was made in the mental health field, particularly for peer support. Rockland State Hospital in New York is one of the most well-known examples at the forefront of the modern peer support movement. During the 1940s, hospital employees worked to form support groups for those living with mental health conditions with the hope that the support they could offer one another after being released would improve their outcomes (Anderson, 1998). Those patients later went on to found Fountain House, the model for today's drop-in centers (Beard, 1978).

In the United States, the 1960s and 1970s saw radical changes in the way in which those living with mental health conditions were understood and treated. Along with advancement in psychiatry and psychology, more concerted efforts were being made to humanize treatment and learn more about the biological and social components of mental health disorders. Part of the growth in the field can be attributed to the advances in medicine. Significantly, it is during this same period that the movements for civil and economic equality were advancing globally. In the United States, the Civil Rights, Black Power, women's rights, and lesbian, gay, bisexual, transgender, queer/questioning-plus (LGBTQ+) movements were gaining power and authority.

It was during this period that important policies and legislation were passed in the United States that better reflected the needs of those receiving services in the behavioral health space. Notably, the Community Mental Health Centers Act (1963) enabled widespread deinstitutionalization of people living within mental health asylums and established community mental health centers (CMHCs). These CMHCs are also the same organizations that typically use peers to provide services to those just beginning their recovery journey.

Additionally, around the world, the former colonial power structure was rapidly coming to an end; nations throughout Africa, South and Central America, and Asia were winning their hard-earned freedom and independence. It was during this fight for equality, across all socioeconomic status (SES), cultural, and racial differences, that the notion of equality and equity in all forms should perhaps be embraced. It was also during these times that, in 1972, the Madness News Network began to publish, advocating for the rights, dignity, and self-expression of mental health patients. The Conference on Human Rights and Against Psychiatric Oppression, first held in 1973, became an annual opportunity to discuss the importance of humane treatment of those seeking mental health services (Corrigan et al., 2024).

OVERVIEW OF PRESENT-DAY PEER SUPPORT SERVICES

Peer support has proliferated over the past 50 years and has become recognized as an important component of mental health and wellness. In the modern-day concept of peers and peerness, a peer can identify with a range of behavioral health conditions from mental illness to substance use. Moreover, peers themselves often come from various racial, educational, ethnic, SES, gender, and gender identity backgrounds (Cronise et al., 2016). The beautiful aspect of being a peer is the ability to be intersectional and embrace all aspects of the self while working with clients. Within this space, those working in peer support generally falls into two categories: (a) informal support and (b) formal or professional peer support. Each is discussed next.

Informal Peer Services

Informal peer support, usually in the form of mutual support or self-help groups, was created to address a variety of issues often overlooked by formal care systems (Lieberman, 1990). These groups offer voluntary, mutual assistance for common needs, life challenges, and personal growth (Katz & Bender, 1976). Typically, free and nonclinician led, these groups provide hope, information, and opportunities for making social connections with those who have similar life experiences. Notable examples include Recovery International, GROW, Schizophrenia & Psychosis Action Alliance,

Double Trouble in Recovery, and Alcoholics Anonymous. Self-help groups range from informal gatherings to highly organized groups with guiding principles and literature. Self-help group attendees report reductions in symptoms, increased quality of life, and enhanced self-esteem (Markowitz, 2015). Ongoing participation appears linked to better outcomes (Markowitz, 2015; Pistrang et al., 2008).

These groups, now using online platforms like Facebook, YouTube, and Zoom, provide high anonymity, reducing social repercussions and facilitating the sharing of sensitive information (Krentzman, 2021). Online support has been beneficial for those lacking local groups, lacking transportation, or facing physical constraints; such support has expanded significantly, especially during the COVID-19 pandemic, and offers both public and private groups that require an application for membership (Fortuna et al., 2022). Self-help groups, especially those that operate in an online-only capacity, are especially proliferating in low- and middle-income countries, making mental health support more accessible.

One-on-one self-help, often arising informally from group connections, includes sponsorship in 12-step models, which has been shown to reduce substance use and enhance personal growth for both sponsors and sponsored party (McGovern et al., 2022). Although research on individual peer support for mental health is limited, the World Health Organization (2019) has provided comprehensive guidelines on this topic.

Formal or Professional Peer Services

Professional peer services, which are delivered by individuals with lived mental illness experience, differ from self-help groups in that peer providers are serving in a professional, often paid, role, and services are more unidirectional (rather than mutual). In 2010, with the passing of the Patient Protection and Affordable Care Act, Medicaid began allowing peer services to be billed (Ostrow et al., 2017), greatly expanding possibilities for the formalization of peer support. Peer professionals now work in a variety of settings, providing services around health, substance use, employment, crisis, outreach, and advocacy (Corrigan, Talluri, & Shah, 2022). Nationwide, at least 37% of mental health agencies have peer support available (Videka et al., 2019), and states have developed credentialing mechanism for peer support providers (Voss et al., 2022). Categories of formal peer services include peer-run services, peer partnerships, and peer employees, varying mainly by the extent of control peers have over administration and decision making of service provision (Clay et al., 2005).

The United States has certified peers in all 50 states. Each state has varying requirements to become certified, but most require at a minimum a high school diploma or equivalent and specific training on mental health (Voss et al., 2022). Illinois is one of the states leading the charge on the professionalization of peers. The state has invested significant sums for the creation of more than 10 state-funded training programs to support peers in becoming certified to provide services in both mental health and substance use disorder. Once a peer has successfully completed the requirements, they are able to bill health insurers for their services and work as providers of mental health and substance use services (Illinois Certification Board, 2024).

The National Association of Peer Supporters (NAPS), founded in 2004, has played a significant role in the professionalization of peers across the United States (see https://www.peersupportworks.org). The nonprofit organization provides support and resources to peer supporters of all professional levels to help them become leaders in their field and provide services to the millions of people across the country who are struggling with mental health conditions or substance use disorder. The NAPS' Global Peer Support Celebration Day increases the visibility of peers in the mental health space and offers an opportunity for advocating for the notions that living well in recovery is possible and likely with necessary support and treatment options (Global Peer Support Celebration Day Committee, n.d.).

Peer-Run Services and Partnerships

Planned and managed entirely by individuals with mental illness, peer-run services adhere to principles of choice and peer control (Fortuna et al., 2022; Ostrow & Hayes, 2015). Examples include drop-in centers, which offer socializing opportunities for those living with mental health conditions, and peer-run respite services that offer a range of activities and crisis alternatives. Comprehensive services may cover employment, housing, benefits acquisition, care coordination, advocacy, crisis services, and psychoeducation (Cook et al., 2020; del Vecchio, 2022). Warm lines provide peer-staffed telephone support, reducing the burden on crisis hotlines (Fortuna et al., 2022). These programs also engage in advocacy, research, and education and are funded by government grants, private foundations, and fees (Ostrow & Hayes, 2015). Positive outcomes of peer-operated services include improved quality of life, reduced hospitalizations, and increased employment and program satisfaction (Swarbrick, 2011; Swarbrick et al., 2016).

Peer partnerships involve shared responsibilities between peers and non-peers. In contrast to peer-operated services, peer partnerships are somewhat less egalitarian. The *clubhouse model* is a notable example; it emphasizes community integration and standardization through fidelity measures and accreditation (McKay et al., 2018). Review by McKay and colleagues has shown benefits in employment, hospitalization reduction, and quality of life within clubhouses.

Peer Employees

Peer employees, individuals with lived experience of mental illness hired in peer-specific roles, offer unique perspectives, coping strategies, and engagement benefits (Fortuna et al., 2022). Challenges include boundary issues, stigma, and acceptance by professional staff (Bellamy et al., 2017; Firmin et al., 2019; Voss et al., 2022). Peer support, continued mental health treatment, supervisory support, and training can all be helpful support strategies in the face of these challenges (Abraham et al., 2021; Forbes et al., 2022; Jenkins et al., 2020). However, some clients may distrust peer employees or feel they are influenced by professional biases (Gillard, 2019). Extensive literature has indicated that peer employee services yield at least modest improvements in symptoms, recovery, and functioning, particularly for individuals with severe mental illness (Lyons et al., 2021; Smit et al., 2022; White et al., 2020). Studies have shown that peer services are at least as effective as those provided by nonpeers with similar training: Peer services have with structured interventions in well-defined roles that demonstrate the most positive effects (Bellamy et al., 2017). Although methodological limitations exist, the evidence has suggested that peer services are beneficial and often enhance hope, recovery, empowerment, and quality of life.

Peer Professionals and the Power of Self-Disclosure

The key to being a peer is a willingness to disclose one's own personal lived experience with a mental health or substance use condition. This critical difference between peers and other mental health service providers offers an important yet necessary distinction. In the past, before the professionalization of peer supporters, self-disclosure of personal mental health challenges was seen as a controversial issue within the realm of mental health (Berg et al., 2020). In the process of disclosing, peers tell their lived experience story in a variety of settings. Disclosure can take many forms: from discussing their full story for an hour at an advocacy event to sharing a piece of their story in a 5-minute conversation with a client. Disclosure is the act of the peer sharing their own lived experience story with others, especially those living in recovery and receiving services. This is done to connect with the clients they serve while also offering advice and hope. In sharing their story, professional peers are able to demonstrate the variety of skills and techniques they have used to maintain recovery, while they also impart this knowledge to their clients.

Peers disclose their stories to support their clients to make informed decisions about their lives. This critical aspect of the peer role allows clients to better understand the myriad choices available to them while living in recovery. Because peers are increasingly in roles of authority and power in CMHCs and medical settings, the use of SDM regarding issues of harm reduction and goal setting is pivotal to supporting clients to enter and maintain recovery.

In general, those who work in the mental health profession often voice concerns about self-disclosure; there can be legitimate worry about the effect that self-disclosure can have on their job opportunities and their perception in the workplace (Byrne et al., 2022). Interestingly, this concern is of paramount importance despite that many mental health professionals acknowledge that they have lived experience outside of their professional roles (Repper & Carter, 2011).

Despite this, strides have been made in the field to allow professionals to disclose their lived experience when it might support their clients. The use of disclosure in this context would be appropriate. This disclosure provides an opportunity for the peer and client to connect and learn from past experiences. Professional peers serve as living examples of recovery and hope that living with a mental health challenge or a substance use challenge does not have to define them. Peer professionals who hold jobs demonstrate that it is possible to live a full life and earn a living even when dealing with symptoms of mental illness or substance use disorder. Seeing someone like themselves provides clients with an opportunity to learn and grow in their own recovery in the hope that they can one day live their lives on their own terms. Hope is indeed one of the many facets in peer support interventions (Fortuna et al., 2019), and fostering hope in the recovery model is an important part of a peer's role is assisting someone in their own lived experience journey.

However, although disclosure is a vital part of the peer role, it is also one that comes with some of the most difficulties. One of the many common questions and concerns that arise from peer supporters is how to disclose their stories and how to know whether the client is ready to hear said story. Importantly, professional peers disclose purely on the basis of supporting clients and helping them move forward in their recovery process.

What can be gleaned from existing research on mental health providers showcases areas of concern with regard to the relationship dynamics between the service provider and the service recipient. However, unlike the traditional therapist model, professional peers are in a mentorship role. They serve as guides in the recovery process as someone who has lived through it and have been able to move past the most challenging circumstances to live well in recovery.

And although disclosing their own lived experience is key to the peer role, some challenges exist. Notably, existing research (Marino et al., 2016) has shown that one of the problems with disclosure is the potential complication of the relationship between the service provider and the service recipient. Professional peers must be especially careful when working with clients because they may be seen as friends rather than support professionals. Maintaining boundaries as a peer is a way to reduce the issue of dual roles and the complication of the professional relationship with clients.

However, disclosure is still a somewhat taboo topic in mental health. Peers are able to traverse this issue and provide support in a way that offers clients a sense of normalcy in their experience in knowing that they are not alone with their struggles. This, in effect, can create a more positive experience for those seeking services, assist with the reduction of stigma, and improve the overall understanding of the importance of disclosure (Byrne et al., 2022).

Evidence-Based Peer Practices

With the proliferation of peer services in past decades, a number of evidence-based peer-led practices have emerged. Selected practices and modalities are summarized in Table 5.1. Some of the evidence-based practices, such as harm reduction, have been borrowed by peers from traditional mental health and substance use practices; others have been developed by and for peers. Peer-developed practices outlined in Table 5.1 include peer health navigation; peer support groups; Wellness Recovery Action Plan (WRAP); Whole Health Action Management; and Honest, Open, Proud (HOP). In still other cases (e.g., assertive community treatment, Individual Placement and Support), peers have joined existing interdisciplinary teams to provide evidence-based services in a team model. Most of these services are provided in formal or professional settings; however, peer support groups, which are arguably the most widespread, are often provided informally. The diversity of peer-provided services is reflected in Table 5.1.

SHARED DECISION MAKING AND PEER SUPPORT

According to the Agency for Healthcare Research and Quality (AHRQ, 2014), SDM involves a patient and health provider engaging in dialogue to jointly make a specific health decision. This dialogue should incorporate medical

TABLE 5.1. Evidence-Based Practices in Peer Support

Practice	Description	Reference
Peer health navigation	Services provided in the community to help people navigate the complexities of obtaining mental and physical health care and self-management	Mullen et al. (2023) Corrigan, Razzano, et al. (2022)
Peer support/ mutual support groups	Semistructured, peer-led support groups (in-person or virtual) to discuss mental health or substance use topics	Lyons et al. (2021) Tracy & Wallace (2016)
Harm reduction	A health approach that helps people identify risk or harms and reduce these harms without the requirement of total abstinence or adherence to recommended treatments	Chang et al. (2021) Mercer et al. (2021)
ACT	Intensive, team-based, case management services provided to people living in community settings in which peers are members of the team	Abufarsakh et al. (2023)
WRAP	Structured, peer-led group and workbook with goal of creating a comprehensive recovery plan	Canacott et al. (2019)
WHAM	Structured, peer-led group that focuses holistically on health self-management	Cook et al. (2020)
IPS	Intensive team-based services to help people obtain and maintain employment, often including a peer team member	Bond et al. (2020)
HOP	A peer-led strategic disclosure and antistigma intervention to consider the pros and cons of sharing lived experiences of mental health challenges	Rüsch & Kösters (2021)

Note. ACT = assertive community treatment; WRAP = Wellness Recovery Action Planning; WHAM = Whole Health Action Management; IPS = Individual Placement and Support; HOP = Honest, Open, Proud.

or research evidence, the patient's preferences and values, and the provider's professional knowledge. Because peers traditionally have not been considered medical providers, they were not initially considered as playing a role in the SDM implementation (Zisman-Ilani & Byrne, 2023). However, with the growth of the peer support movement has come greater expansion into this important role, and the underlying principles align. In this section, we consider SDM by peer providers related to health decisions regarding physical illness, mental illness, and domains of wellness broadly (e.g., work, spiritual, social). We begin this section by highlighting some SDM interventions that involve peers.

Specific Shared Decision Making Interventions Involving Peers

The most researched and implemented peer-involved SDM intervention (Thomas et al., 2023), called CommonGround, was developed by Pat Deegan (2010) using codesign. CommonGround is a tool to guide SDM between prescribers and users using a software-guided system. Peer staff are part of the SDM team, helping the client to adopt SDM practices. In CommonGround, the client arrives early to their psychiatry appointment, and a peer helps them use the SDM software. The software generates a report that is then used to guide SDM discussion during the prescribing appointment. Peers are again available after the prescribing appointment to provide support. The software program itself includes a survey about recovery, symptoms, use of medications, concerns, goal for the appointment, goals for psychiatric medicine, and overall wellness goals. CommonGround has also been adapted and evaluated abroad (Yamaguchi et al., 2017). A similar program, SDM Digital Intake, is administered at clinics specific to people with depression, anxiety, or personality disorders (Metz et al., 2018). With assistance from a peer, clients complete a series of digital modules about their needs and preferences before beginning services.

Other SDM models have involved peers along with a more extensive team of providers. Paudel and colleagues (2018) created a model involving a psychiatrist, nurse, and peer worker that includes group sessions to prepare clients for SDM, including goal setting and psychoeducation. Just Do You, an SDM intervention aimed at emerging adults, includes sessions led jointly by peers and a clinician that are focused on psychoeducation, motivational interviewing, and personal narratives (Munson et al., 2021). Additionally, an SDM intervention aimed at self-management and care planning calls for case managers and peers to colead skills groups and engage in collaborative care planning (Lawn et al., 2007).

Shared Ideals Between Shared Decision Making and Peer Support

Peer support and SDM share similar ideals because both were developed to combat coercion and lack of choices for clients (Zisman-Ilani & Byrne, 2023). Figure 5.1 shows the 12 core values of peer support, as described by NAPS (2013). Among these values are three that are particularly relevant to

FIGURE 5.1. Core Values From Practice Guidelines of the National Association of Peer Supporters

Voluntary	**Hopeful**	**Open Minded**	**Empathetic**
Respectful	**Facilitate Change**	**Honest and Direct**	**Mutual and Reciprocal**
Equally Share Power	**Strengths-Focused**	**Transparent**	**Person-Driven**

Note. Data from National Association of Peer Supporters (2013).

the practice of SDM: (a) power sharing (similar to equally sharing power), (b) person-driven, and (c) open minded.

Power Sharing

To come to a decision that is truly a shared one, the health provider must be mindful of their inherent social power relative to the client. A medical doctor is one of the most revered professional positions in our society and often has the power to grant or deny access to medications, medical tests, procedures, or insurance coverage for these services based on their expert opinions. Therefore, they are entering the SDM relationship at a considerable power advantage over a patient, who may often hesitate to be critical of their knowledge, opinions, or authority. Moreover, this power differential can be even more pronounced for patients who come from underserved and disenfranchised backgrounds, such as communities of color; lesbian, gay, bisexual, transgender, queer/questioning-plus (LGBTQ+); people with disabilities; lower levels of formal education; and low SES. For true SDM to occur, a medical provider must be willing and able to share power with the client to thoroughly discuss their preferences and come to a decision that aligns with those preferences and needs. Sharing power with clients requires providers to openly acknowledge that the client is the ultimate decision-maker for their treatment and recovery goals. As such, they are experts in their own experience, and providers should strive to serve as a support person for clients rather than an authoritarian expert.

In peer support, peer providers also strive to share power in the relationship with the clients as a core value. Although the initial power differential between client and peer provider may be inherently lower than that between doctor and patient, these power differentials still exist and should be explicitly discussed and monitored within the relationship to achieve the highest quality rapport.

Person-Driven

A person-driven approach is essential to peer support, which recognizes that the person knows what is best for themselves, and the peer supporter helps them to that end. Similarly, at its core, SDM is an essential part to the recovery journey (Alguera-Lara et al., 2017). An important tenet of SDM is taking the client's preferences into account (Thomas et al., 2023). Clients have reported lower levels of symptoms and higher levels of satisfaction with life as a result of their perceived notions of agency and informed decision-making capabilities (Pfeiffer et al., 2011). Although the health provider can present information about health conditions and procedures, in SDM, they must converse with the client about their preferences and about how a health decision might affect their life. SDM allows those living with mental health challenges to have agency to make final decisions about what is best for their own lives, treatment, and long-term care for the health conditions in which they live. This is based on the notion of values-based practice (Berg et al., 2020). In this model, the providers of services lay out the needed information for the service recipient to make the decision (Alguera-Lara et al., 2017). In this manner, patients must feel comfortable discussing their needs and rationale behind their choices with the service providers. Service providers should also be comfortable being open to the ambivalence and potential lack of interest in treatment options exhibited by clients.

Open Mindedness

Providing peer support requires an open mind about the choices a client might make. Although a peer support professional may have been tremendously helped by antidepressant medication, they must not assume that antidepressants will be the proverbial magic bullet for every client. They should keep an open mind about client choices and maintain a nonjudgmental stance. SDM also requires this type of open-mindedness to facilitate the collaboration needed. Open mindedness will also help reduce power differentials between provider and client.

SHARED DECISION MAKING VERSUS SUPPORTED DECISION MAKING

The term *supported decision making*, which originated with the disability rights movement, describes the provision of general support to individuals with cognitive disabilities during the decision-making process (Simmons & Gooding, 2017). Health care providers or family members might assume that individuals with cognitive disabilities, including psychiatric disabilities, are incapable of making decisions and commandeer the decision making on their behalf. In supported decision making, autonomous decision making is viewed as a human right, much like the right to live in the least restrictive environment or the right to public education. Individuals with psychiatric disability are often provided with supported employment services to help find and keep employment. In a similar way, supported decision making can allow individuals to enact important life choices (e.g., housing, finances, hospitalization) beyond medical decisions. Whereas SDM calls for a joint process in which at least two individuals (usually health provider and patient) reach a decision, supported decision making recognizes the client's ability to make decisions and could reduce power imbalance inherent in SDM (e.g., physician is recognized as the expert). Decision making enacted in the context of peer support more closely resembles that of supported decision making. Therefore, some might prefer this terminology. Supported decision making, when enacted by peers, might challenge issues of power imbalance and stigma. Supported decision making in recent years has increased, involving areas such as advance directives and advocacy services (Arstein-Kerslake et al., 2017; Francis et al., 2024; Gooding, 2013; Minkowitz, 2010), which are in the scope of practice of peer professionals.

We maintain that peers can best support client decision making in two ways: (a) by helping clients enact SDM in conjunction with other health care providers and (b) by engaging clients in SDM around holistic life decisions that affect health and well-being. We discuss each of these in depth and provide examples of these from the field.

Peer Enactment of SDM in Collaboration With Health Care Providers

By the nature of their relationship to the client, peers are uniquely positioned to collaborate with health care providers (e.g., physicians, psychiatrists, nurses, therapists) in implementing SDM (Schladitz et al., 2023). For example, peers might assist clients in preparing for meetings with health care providers, join decision-making sessions with health care providers, or assist with the logistics of implementing shared decisions. In their examination of 10 systematic reviews of 100 mental health–specific SDM studies, Chmielowska and colleagues (2023) found that most SDM programs focused on implementing SDM in dyadic relationships (most often patients–clients) rather than through a team model. However, team models that include peers are becoming more common (see Thomas et al., 2023). Peers bring several important aspects to the practice of SDM: trust and rapport, emotional support and motivation, communication and self-advocacy support, and information and practical support.

Trust and Rapport

One of the benefits of using peers is their knowledge of the lived experience with mental health challenges. They can connect with clients because they have struggled with and survived similar experiences. Additionally, peers' focus on recovery is a departure from the traditional clinical model, which focuses on diagnosis and symptom reduction. Peers often understand at a visceral level the myriad nuances of living with a mental health challenge. As peers, they use recovery-oriented language that focuses on holistic life goals rather than illness or symptoms. Because of the historical lack of respect for people with mental health challenges and the sometimes degrading treatment they have received, allowing clients to openly communicate their concerns requires time, patience, and understanding. Often, it is the peer professionals who provide this bridge level of support to help clients communicate with therapists and other providers. Having a peer to support clients through SDM can help them feel more trust in the process and become more engaged in SDM, especially when peer supporters share their own experiences with decision making (Thomas et al., 2023).

Emotional Support and Motivation

In SDM, peers can provide needed emotional support to help them process feelings around potentially life-altering decisions. This emotional support can help clients to further build their self-efficacy in making decisions (Thomas et al., 2023). Peers can increase the motivation of clients to engage in decision making through modeling and encouragement. When a peer supporter talks about their experiences with SDM or asks the client to share their own experiences or opinions on the topic, this may activate self-determination that another health provider might not be able to elicit.

Communication and Self-Advocacy Support

Peers can facilitate communication between the client and other providers (e.g., psychiatrists) and support clients in advocating for their needs in the decision-making process (Thomas et al., 2023). Peers serve as a vital guide on the recovery journey. Instead of holding the title of clinician or doctor, they provide a bridge to wellness even amid what may be heartbreaking despair or frustration with the symptoms of mental illness. Their role often leads to more egalitarian communication and a relationship based on shared experiences rather than a superficially imposed hierarchy. Often, clients feel more comfortable talking to peers about their challenges because of the less stringent professional distance and because peers have been in similar situations. Similarly, supporting self-advocacy is a chief issue for peers. As such, peers who are respected contributors to the SDM treatment team are critical in helping clients reclaim their power. With this support, clients can then work toward living out their ideal recovery-oriented journey.

Information and Practical Support

Peers can also help with information and practice supports (Thomas et al., 2023). Peers have made many of their own decisions related to mental or physical health and have important knowledge of the community and treatment options that they can provide clients. Peers can also aid clients in the logistics of using decision aids or decision-making tools. Peers can assist clients in enacting decisions that are made via SDM by helping them navigate health care or social services to get their needs met (e.g., helping them find a specialist, getting a second opinion, obtaining health insurance coverage). An example of practical support has emerged in the area of social prescribing. Psychiatrists who believe their patients might benefit from more social support can use an SDM process to prescribe social services that both the peer supporter and the patient can decide on and that a peer implements (Zisman-Ilani et al., 2023).

Peer-Led Shared Decision Making About Health and Life Decisions

Although in practice peer professionals are often engaging with clients around decision making, it is not always done in a structured way or labeled as SDM. Peer-led decision support might involve coaching guidance, psychoeducation, motivational strategies or use of specific decision aids or tools (Thomas et al., 2023). Table 5.1 showed a variety of existing peer practices that incorporate decision-making processes—some more explicitly than others. Peer support groups, for example, focus on social and emotional support; however, group members often assist one another in decision making. On the more explicit side, WRAP is a peer-facilitated course that provides attendees with workbooks that guide them in completing a recovery plan. Many activities in the workbook require decisions on coping strategies, wellness routines, and social supports, among others. In addition, HOP is a peer-led group that guides decision making around mental health disclosure. Implicit in these programs is the assumption that decisions are driven by the client's wants, needs, and abilities. Peer-facilitated decision-making programs beyond those highlighted in Table 5.1 are also proliferating. For example, a group of researchers and people with lived experience developed a decision-support tool for peer professionals to enhance SDM in selecting mental health technology (Mbao et al., 2021). The tool helps clients consider aspects of each technology (e.g., usability, costs, accessibility, privacy or security) when selecting phone apps, virtual reality, video games, or social media. Another example of peer-facilitated decision making is the CHOICE (Choices about Healthcare Options Informed by Client Experiences and Expectations) pilot program in Australia, which focuses on decision making for youth with mental illness (Simmons et al., 2018).

Given the vast scope of peer support services, Table 5.2 outlines opportunities for shared or supported decision making within the various domains of peer support. Although this is not an exhaustive list, the table organizes peer support into nine domains: (a) health promotion; (b) illness self-management; (c) crisis services; (d) employment and education; (e) substance use; (f) housing; (g) forensic or transition services; (h) advocacy, antistigma, and storytelling or disclosure; and (i) social participation. The questions in the second column suggest areas for the development of explicit tools or aids or more informal conversation starters for a supported or shared decision-making process between peer and client. For example, a client might mention to their peer provider that they never want to go to Hospital X ever again. This could initiate a conversation with the peer provider about alternatives to hospitalization, transportation options to other hospitals, or more extensive crisis planning. Similarly, a SDM tool (e.g., worksheet, phone app) could be created to guide decision making around mental health crisis.

To further demonstrate SDM in peer practice, Exhibit 5.1 depicts a dialogue between a fictional client, Amy, and their peer support worker, Manuel. In this scenario, Amy is considering telling their supervisor about their depression so that they can request workplace accommodation but is worried about potential negative implications. Manuel talks Amy through the decision, providing emotional support and helping them role-play possible scenarios to build their self-efficacy. Note that Manuel does not advise Amy about what they should decide or even pressure Amy to make any decision at all during the discussion.

Manuel's conversation with Amy provided a cursory example of shared decision making (SDM). Those who wish to begin incorporating SDM into peer work might benefit from the structure of a model. The Agency for Healthcare Research and Quality (AHRQ) SHARE Model of SDM (see Table 5.3), provides five steps to guide the process: (a) S: Seek the client's participation; (b) H: Help the client explore options and the pros and cons of each option; (c) A: Assess the client's values and preferences; (d) R: Reach a decision with your client; and (e) E: Evaluate your client's decision.

TABLE 5.2. Opportunities for Shared Decision Making in Peer Services

Service domain	Opportunities for SDM
Health promotion and wellness	• What healthy activities might enhance my life? • How might I be more active? • How can I improve my eating habits? • What activities might enhance my life? • How might spirituality contribute to my wellness? • What are my recovery goals?
Illness self-management	• When do I want to see a doctor or specialist? • How do I want to manage my medications? • What lifestyle choices would help me manage my health? • What self-care activities might I engage in? • What are treatment options for me?
Crisis services	• What hospital do I want to go to if I am in crisis? How do I want to get there? • What are my alternatives to hospitalization? • What other supports can I use? • How do I want to communicate with others during periods of mental health instability? • What advance directives do I want in place?
Employment and education	• What are my priority career or educational goals? • What are first steps toward career and educational goals? • Do I want to pursue a new employment opportunity, promotion, or career change?
Substance use	• Do I want to reduce or stop using substances? What are supports and options for doing this?
Housing	• How can I improve my current living situation? • How do housing options fit with my recovery goals?
Forensic or transition services	• What supports do I want in place during the transition from incarceration to the community?
Advocacy, antistigma, and storytelling or disclosure	• Do I want to, or how do I want to, be involved in mental health advocacy? • How might I challenge the stigma of mental illness? • What do I want to share about my experiences and in what context of my life? • How can I advocate for myself?
Social participation	• In what ways do I want my social life to change? • What community activities might I participate in? • Do I want to enhance my relationships with others? Do I want to pursue a new relationship? Do I want to end a relationship?

Note. SDM = shared decision making.

EXHIBIT 5.1. Peer-Led Shared Decision Making: Amy and Manuel

Here, we present a sample dialogue between Amy, a service user, and their peer support worker, Manuel.

AMY: Hi, Manuel. I've been feeling really anxious lately, and I think it might be because I'm considering telling my boss about my depression. I'm not sure if that's the right thing to do.

MANUEL: Hi there. I'm glad you brought this up. Deciding whether to talk about that at work can be challenging. Can you tell me more about what's making you consider this now?

AMY: Well, I've been having a hard time keeping up with my tasks. I feel like if my boss knew, they might understand why I'm not performing at my best and maybe even offer some support or accommodations.

MANUEL: That makes sense. I know when I was struggling at work when my symptoms first got bad, it was hard for me to focus. I was also scared about what people might think of me if I requested accommodations. However, it was really important for me to do it so I could get the support I needed. Have you thought about what kind of support you might need from your boss?

AMY: Yes, I think having a more flexible schedule or the ability to work from home occasionally would really help me manage my symptoms better.

MANUEL: Those seem like reasonable requests. It's good to have a clear idea of what you need. I know when I requested accommodations, they really helped! And it was super helpful to know I had a boss on my side. Do you think your boss would be helpful?

AMY: I think so. My boss has always seemed understanding, but I'm still worried. What if they react negatively, or it changes how they see me?

MANUEL: It's natural to worry about that. It helps to prepare for the conversation. That way, you can think about how to explain your situation clearly and what specific support you're asking for. Would you like to role-play this conversation together to feel better about going into the conversation with them?

AMY: That sounds like a good idea. I could use the practice.

MANUEL: Great. Let's start with you explaining your situation to me as if I'm your boss. Take your time.

AMY: Okay, um. . . . "Hi, I wanted to talk to you about something, Manuel. I've been dealing with depression, and it's been affecting my work. I'm seeking treatment, but I think having a more flexible schedule or the option to work from home occasionally could really help me manage my workload better."

MANUEL: That's a good start. You're being honest and direct. How do you think your boss might respond?

AMY: Maybe they'll ask how exactly it's been affecting my work or if there's anything else they can do to help.

MANUEL: Yes, so let's talk about and practice some more how you might respond to follow-up questions.

EXHIBIT 5.1. Peer-Led Shared Decision Making: Amy and Manuel (*Continued*)

Manuel and Amy continue with discussion and role plays for another 15 minutes.

MANUEL: How are you feeling now?

AMY: I feel a bit more prepared, but I'm still nervous.

MANUEL: That's completely understandable. Remember: It's okay to be nervous. You're taking an important step for your well-being. If you decide to go through with this, you can always follow up with me to discuss how it went and any next steps. And if you decide not to tell them right now, that's okay too. It's your decision.

AMY: Thanks, Manuel. I really appreciate your support. I'll think about it some more, and maybe we can talk about it again next session?

MANUEL: Of course. I'm here to support you no matter what you decide.

Note. Case examples in this book are hypothetical.

TABLE 5.3. Activating Questions for Each Stage of the Agency for Healthcare Research and Quality's SHARE Model of Shared Decision Making

SDM steps in the SHARE model	Sample activating questions
Seek client's participation	• One of the items you listed on your wellness plan is having more social connections. Are you interested in discussing some options for developing your social network?
Help client explore options and the pros and cons of each option	• What kinds of social activities might you be interested in? • What are the pros and cons of joining a book club?
Assess client's values and preferences	• What is important to you in a friendship? • What kind of social contact are you most comfortable with?
Reach a decision with your client	• Are you ready to make a decision on this now or do you need more time? • What option is best for you? • What more information do you need?
Evaluate your client's decision	• Is it okay if we talk about this more next week to see how it's going?

Note. SDM = shared decision making. Adapted from *The SHARE Approach: Essential Steps of Shared Decision-Making: Quick Reference Guide* (p. 2), by Agency for Healthcare Research and Quality, 2014 (https://archive.ahrq.gov/health-literacy/professional-training/shared-decision/tools/share-tool1.pdf). In the public domain.

The second column of Table 5.3 suggests questions that might encourage clients to engage with peer support at each step. For example, peers might seek their clients' participation by asking, "Are you interested in discussing some options for developing your social network?" Note that the AHRQ model was created for use with medical decisions in health care and may need to be adapted for a specific setting or purpose; nevertheless, it can provide a useful framework for ensuring SDM is infused throughout the entire process.

Benefits of Peer Involvement in Shared Decision Making

There are a number of purported benefits to peer-led decision-making programs, including enhanced engagement in treatment, improved functioning, enhanced perceptions of decision making, and a reduction in decisional conflict (Thomas et al., 2023). Peer professionals who provide decision supports also benefit in terms of self-efficacy and personal–professional growth. Moreover, as the barriers to enter the field of peer support are lower than for clinician positions, the time frame to enter into the workforce as a peer professional is quicker, allowing peer professionals to enter the field and bring principles of SDM to fruition as well as fill needed gaps in mental health services that complement therapy and more traditional psychological services.

Peer-led decision-making interventions can also lead to transformation of systems. Rooted in the value system of peer support is the idea that peers, both professional and voluntary, use their shared experiences and agency to advance the recovery journey and process. This, by extension, is applied to organizations that use peer support and their ability to effectively implement peer services. Through fully integrating peers and acknowledging the peer experience as a professional level of expertise, treatment teams can provide holistic support to service recipients (Wu et al., 2023). Ultimately, full integration of peers into the clinical model best serves clients.

Once integrated into the organization, peers may have the opportunity to grow and flourish in their roles and in supporting clients to achieve their objectives. Not only is this an important part of development as an organization, but it also demonstrates the importance of recovery and the recovery journey to the clients they serve. No longer are clients willing to be "othered"; rather, they are clients just like any other deserving of respect and care that is in alignment with their culture, values, and belief systems.

Research has noted that clients typically prefer to work with providers who are racially and ethnically congruent to themselves (Alang, 2019). This may be because of having less need to explain cultural nuances or background information and less concern about bias and racism. Peers are often providing services in community mental health settings and reflect the communities in which they serve, with many identifying as people of color, LGBTQ+, or both. As such, there is a level of understanding relating to community and shared experiences.

Potential Challenges of Peer Involvement in Shared Decision Making

Although peer support has a long history of user-driven decision making, there are multiple challenges to implementation of decisional supports or incorporation of peers into more traditional SDM. Professional peers' abilities to provide support as part of the team may be questioned by other mental health professionals. It is not uncommon for those peers to be relegated to tasks that are unsuited to their expertise and training. Peers are often paid significantly less than their clinician colleagues and sometimes work in environments that have significantly higher caseloads than their colleagues. As such, although peers may be increasing in number in the behavioral health field, there is still substantial stigma and bias against them (Myrick & del Vecchio, 2016). Mental health professionals may have concerns about peer professionals' recovery, chiefly that a relapse or slip in their mental health may occur and result in regression in their recovery process.

An additional challenge to the shared decision-making process is the stigma that inevitably comes with including those who are often seen by the medical community as having less ability to take part in their health care decisions. This is especially true for those living with serious mental illnesses, such as schizophrenia and bipolar disorder. Doubly so, professional peers who have these and other conditions may live with the ramifications of stigmatized mental health conditions and face it as patients and in the workplace (Thomas et al., 2023).

Once peers have obtained the requisite level of organizational and professional support, other challenges remain in the shared decision-making process. Chief among them is the often daunting task of working with clients who are acutely ill (Haugom et al., 2023). In these cases, there is legitimate concern about the efficacy and feasibility of sharing decision-making power and authority with a client who may not have the mental capacity to make decisions in their own best interest (Schladitz et al., 2023). Dispute over what constitutes a client "in the right state of mind" can be subjective. Organizations that are overly concerned with risk management may hesitate to endorse client-directed decisions that are potentially harmful to the client (e.g., moving out of a nursing home setting; Francis et al., 2024). Even health providers with intentions of empowerment and self-determination may have difficulty implementing SDM in settings that are inherently controlling and coercive (e.g., prisons, nursing homes; Schladitz et al., 2023).

Interprofessional SDM interventions could also include instances in which peer providers may be asked to provide information or advice beyond their expertise (Cleary et al., 2018). Because of power imbalances, peer providers may be pressured to go along with a decision they do not agree with or one that is not client driven or recovery oriented (Cleary et al., 2018; Thomas et al., 2023). Disparities may exist in resource allocation to members of the team, or the team may face issues with integration (Thomas et al., 2023). Overall, limited resources and knowledge exist to implement decision-making interventions in mental health (Francis et al., 2024), which further complicates these challenges.

FUTURE DIRECTIONS FOR PEER SUPPORT AND SHARED DECISION MAKING

Further development and implementation of SDM in peer support involve three main areas of need: (a) tool or model development, (b) training, and (c) research. With the development of these implementation areas, the field of peer support within SDM can further advance for the benefit of all peers.

Tool Development

Most SDM interventions in mental health have focused on medication decisions and were adapted from medical settings. Most have not been designed for broader health, wellness, and life decision making; thus, there is a need to develop evidence-based SDM intervention for nonclinical services (Zisman-Ilani & Byrne, 2023). Most existing SDM tools are designed to promote dyadic (provider–client) decision making. Tools or models that include peers in prescribed roles within the model or include collaborations with additional support people (e.g., families, friends, partners) in the decision-making process may be preferred for some clients (Chmielowska et al., 2023). To combat challenges with power sharing, mechanisms that encourage peers to disagree with other SDM providers could be built into the models (Zisman-Ilani & Byrne, 2023). As previous models of SDM in peer support have done (e.g., Deegan, 2010), coproduction of SDM tools will be an important practice.

Training

Overall, research shows SDM trainings improve knowledge and skills of training recipients; further, trainings for both peers and clinicians have been feasible and well received (Coates & Clerke, 2020). Trainings may be particularly useful when they are conducted on the use of a specific tool rather than more generally on SDM. Nonpeer clinicians may require training in power sharing to work with peers on SDM intervention teams; likewise, peer providers need training and support in how to communicate around the core values of peer support, voice their opinions, and assist clients in self-advocacy. Peers and nonpeers who engaged in decision making with their clients will also benefit from training in reflexive practice in which providers are encouraged to consider their own biases, attitudes, and actions in relation to others. Although peers share similar experiences with their clients and connect with them based on their experiences, they need to recognize how clients with different worldviews and experiences from their own approach decisions and consider how they can respond in supportive ways when their own worldviews are challenged. Clients will have preferred styles for making decisions that peers may need to accommodate. For example, a peer provider may become frustrated with an adult client who defers to their parent on every decision because the peer provider values a process of systematic and independent decision making. Tools and models should be created or adapted for culture, race or ethnicity, or intersectional identities (Thomas et al., 2023). For instance, an SDM tool meant for Native American men with alcohol use disorder should be developed in collaboration with this group and will have different components than a similar intervention for college students with attention-deficit/hyperactivity disorder.

Research

Relatively few SDM interventions that have been examined through research are completely peer led; therefore, research has been unable to unpack the specific effects on peer professionals within the SDM intervention (Thomas et al., 2023). Although many peer-led interventions include decision-making components, few have evaluated the decision-making approaches or processes separate from the larger intervention. An important part of peer support is sharing stories of discovery and self-disclosure; it remains to be seen what role personal narratives contribute in the context of decision making. Most research outcomes for SDM interventions are medically based (e.g., medication adherence) and do not include outcomes that might be important to clients, such as recovery, stigma, and empowerment (Chmielowska et al., 2023). Research that is done in collaboration with individuals with lived experience of mental health challenges may focus more on client-preferred outcomes of SDM and result in interventions that are more reflective of the lived-experience perspective (Thomas et al., 2023).

CONCLUSION

Historically, peer providers in the behavioral health field have had an important role in promoting the autonomy and self-determination of people with mental illness. In peer support, self-disclosure by peers is an imperative task that allows them to connect with clients on a level of understanding that those who are not peers cannot. Peer support and SDM share important ideals, including sharing power, being person driven, and maintaining an open mind regarding the recovery process.

This chapter has highlighted SDM interventions that involve peer professionals and outlined how some evidence-based practices in peer support include elements of SDM. We also discussed future directions for peer-specific SDM development, training, and research. As peers continue to enter the behavioral health field as professionals with lived experience, they bring valuable insight to the recovery journey and expand opportunities for SDM that can allow clients to feel more comfortable expressing themselves and describing their needs to providers.

REFERENCES

Abraham, K. M., Erickson, P. S., Sata, M. J., & Lewis, S. B. (2021). Job satisfaction and burnout among peer support specialists: The contributions of supervisory mentorship, recovery-oriented workplaces, and role clarity. *Advances in Mental Health, 20*(1), 38–50. https://doi.org/10.1080/18387357.2021.1977667

Abufarsakh, B., Kappi, A., Pemberton, K. M., Williams, L. B., & Okoli, C. T. C. (2023). Substance use outcomes among individuals with severe mental illnesses receiving assertive community treatment: A systematic review. *International Journal of Mental Health Nursing, 32*(3), 704–726. https://doi.org/10.1111/inm.13103

Agency for Healthcare Research and Quality. (2014, April). *The SHARE approach: Essential steps of shared decision-making: Quick reference guide.* https://archive.ahrq.gov/health-literacy/professional-training/shared-decision/tools/share-tool1.pdf

Alang, S. M. (2019). Mental health care among Blacks in America: Confronting racism and constructing solutions. *Health Services Research, 54*(2), 346–355. https://doi.org/10.1111/1475-6773.13115

Alguera-Lara, V., Dowsey, M. M., Ride, J., Kinder, S., & Castle, D. (2017). Shared decision making in mental health: The importance for current clinical practice. *Australasian Psychiatry, 25*(6), 578–582. https://doi.org/10.1177/1039856217734711

Anderson, S. B. (1998). *We are not alone: Fountain House and the development of the clubhouse culture.* Fountain House.

Arstein-Kerslake, A., Watson, J., Browning, M., Martinis, J., & Blanck, P. (2017). Future directions in supported decision-making. *Disability Studies Quarterly, 37*(1). https://doi.org/10.18061/dsq.v37i1.5070

Beard, J. H. (1978). The rehabilitation services of Fountain House. In L. I. Stein & M. A. Test (Eds.), *Alternatives to mental hospital treatment* (pp. 201–208). Plenum Press.

Bellamy, C., Schmutte, T., & Davidson, L. (2017). An update on the growing evidence base for peer support. *Mental Health and Social Inclusion, 21*(3), 161–167. https://doi.org/10.1108/MHSI-03-2017-0014

Berg, H., Bjornestad, J., Våpenstad, E. V., Davidson, L., & Binder, P. E. (2020). Therapist self-disclosure and the problem of shared-decision making. *Journal of Evaluation in Clinical Practice, 26*(2), 397–402. https://doi.org/10.1111/jep.13289

Bond, G. R., Drake, R. E., & Becker, D. R. (2020). An update on individual placement and support. *World Psychiatry, 19*(3), 390–391. https://doi.org/10.1002/wps.20784

Byrne, L., Roennfeldt, H., Davidson, L., Miller, R., & Bellamy, C. (2022). To disclose or not to disclose? Peer workers impact on a culture of safe disclosure for mental health professionals with lived experience. *Psychological Services, 19*(1), 9–18. https://doi.org/10.1037/ser0000555

Canacott, L., Moghaddam, N., & Tickle, A. (2019). Is the Wellness Recovery Action Plan (WRAP) efficacious for improving personal and clinical recovery outcomes? A systematic review and meta-analysis. *Psychiatric Rehabilitation Journal, 42*(4), 372–381. https://doi.org/10.1037/prj0000368

Chang, J., Shelly, S., Busz, M., Stoicescu, C., Iryawan, A. R., Madybaeva, D., de Boer, Y., & Guise, A. (2021). Peer driven or driven peers? A rapid review of peer involvement of people who use drugs in HIV and harm reduction services in low- and middle-income countries. *Harm Reduction Journal, 18*(1), Article 15. https://doi.org/10.1186/s12954-021-00461-z

Chmielowska, M., Zisman-Ilani, Y., Saunders, R., & Pilling, S. (2023). Trends, challenges, and priorities for shared decision making in mental health: The first umbrella review. *The International Journal of Social Psychiatry, 69*(4), 823–840. https://doi.org/10.1177/00207640221140291

Clay, S., Schnell, B., Corrigan, P. W., & Ralph, R. O. (Eds.). (2005). *On our own, together: Peer programs for people with mental illness.* Vanderbilt University Press.

Cleary, M., Raeburn, T., Escott, P., West, S., & Lopez, V. (2018). "Walking the tightrope": The role of peer support workers in facilitating consumers' participation in decision-making. *International Journal of Mental Health Nursing, 27*(4), 1266–1272. https://doi.org/10.1111/inm.12474

Coates, D., & Clerke, T. (2020). Training interventions to equip health care professionals with shared decision-making skills: A systematic scoping review. *The Journal of Continuing Education in the Health Professions, 40*(2), 100–119. https://doi.org/10.1097/CEH.0000000000000289

Community Mental Health Centers Act, Pub. L. No. 88-164, 42 U.S.C. 2689 et seq. (1963). https://www.congress.gov/bill/88th-congress/senate-bill/1576

Cook, J. A., Jonikas, J. A., Burke-Miller, J. K., Hamilton, M., Powell, I. G., Tucker, S. J., Wolfgang, J. B., Fricks, L., Weidenaar, J., Morris, E., & Powers, D. L. (2020).

Whole health action management: A randomized controlled trial of a peer-led health promotion intervention. *Psychiatric Services, 71*(10), 1039–1046. https://doi.org/10.1176/appi.ps.202000012

Corrigan, P. W., Razzano, L., Pashka, N., Ruppert, S., Blaney Rychener, M., Ruiz, A., Kundert, C., & Sheehan, L. (2022). Peer navigators for the health needs of people of color with serious mental illness. *Psychiatric Services, 73*(10), 1182–1185. https://doi.org/10.1176/appi.ps.202100547

Corrigan, P. W., Rüsch, N., Watson, A. C., Kosyluk, K., & Sheehan, L. (2024). *Principles and practice of psychiatric rehabilitation: Promoting recovery and self-determination* (3rd ed.). The Guilford Press.

Corrigan, P. W., Talluri, S. S., & Shah, B. (2022). Formal peer-support services that address priorities of people with psychiatric disabilities: A systematic review. *American Psychologist, 77*(9), 1104–1116. https://doi.org/10.1037/amp0001039

Cronise, R., Teixeira, C., Rogers, E. S., & Harrington, S. (2016). The peer support workforce: Results of a national survey. *Psychiatric Rehabilitation Journal, 39*(3), 211–221. https://doi.org/10.1037/prj0000222

Deegan, P. E. (2010). A web application to support recovery and shared decision making in psychiatric medication clinics. *Psychiatric Rehabilitation Journal, 34*(1), 23–28. https://doi.org/10.2975/34.1.2010.23.28

del Vecchio, P. (2022). Peer service providers as colleagues. In W. E. Sowers, H. L. McQuistion, J. M. Ranz, J. M. Feldman, & P. S. Runnels (Eds.), *Textbook of community psychiatry: American Association for Community Psychiatry* (2nd ed., pp. 525–534). Springer.

Firmin, R. L., Mao, S., Bellamy, C. D., & Davidson, L. (2019). Peer support specialists' experiences of microaggressions. *Psychological Services, 16*(3), 456–462. https://doi.org/10.1037/ser0000297

Forbes, J., Pratt, C., & Cronise, R. (2022). Experiences of peer support specialists supervised by nonpeer supervisors. *Psychiatric Rehabilitation Journal, 45*(1), 54–60. https://doi.org/10.1037/prj0000475

Fortuna, K. L., Ferron, J., Pratt, S. I., Muralidharan, A., Aschbrenner, K. A., Williams, A. M., Deegan, P. E., & Salzer, M. (2019). Unmet needs of people with serious mental illness: Perspectives from certified peer specialists. *Psychiatric Quarterly, 90*(3), 579–586. https://doi.org/10.1007/s11126-019-09647-y

Fortuna, K. L., Solomon, P., & Rivera, J. (2022). An update of peer support/peer provided services underlying processes, benefits, and critical ingredients. *Psychiatric Quarterly, 93*, 571–586. https://doi.org/10.1007/s11126-022-09971-w

Francis, C. J., Johnson, A., & Wilson, R. L. (2024). Supported decision-making interventions in mental healthcare: A systematic review of current evidence and implementation barriers. *Health Expectations, 27*(2), Article e14001. https://doi.org/10.1111/hex.14001

Gillard, S. (2019). Peer support in mental health services: Where is the research taking us, and do we want to go there? *Journal of Mental Health, 28*(4), 341–344. https://doi.org/10.1080/09638237.2019.1608935

Global Peer Support Celebration Day Committee. (n.d.). *Global Peer Support Celebration Day (GPSCD): Toolkit*. National Association of Peer Supporters. https://www.peersupportworks.org/wp-content/uploads/2023/08/Global-Peer-Support-Celebration-Day-Toolkit-202308031542.pdf

Gooding, P. (2013). Supported decision-making: a rights-based disability concept and its implications for mental health law. *Psychiatry, Psychology and Law, 20*(3), 431–451. https://doi.org/10.1080/13218719.2012.711683

Haugom, E. W., Benth, J. Š., Stensrud, B., Stensrud, B., Ruud, T., Calusen, T., & Landheim, A. S. (2023). Shared decision making and associated factors among patients with psychotic disorders: A cross-sectional study. *BMC Psychiatry, 23,* Article 747. https://doi.org/10.1186/s12888-023-05257-y

Himelhoch, M. S., & Shaffer, A. H. (1979). Elizabeth Packard: Nineteenth-century crusader for the rights of mental patients. *Journal of American Studies, 13*(3), 343–375. https://doi.org/10.1017/S0021875800007404

Illinois Certification Board. (2024, July). *The Illinois model for Mental Health Certified Recovery Support Specialist (CRSS*SM*)*. Illinois Alcohol and Other Drug Abuse Professional Certification Association. https://iaodapca.org/Portals/0/PDF/CRSS%20Model%20April%202023.pdf

Jenkins, G. T., Shafer, M. S., & Janich, N. (2020). Critical issues in leadership development for peer support specialists. *Community Mental Health Journal, 56*(6), 1085–1094. https://doi.org/10.1007/s10597-020-00569-9

Katz, A. H., & Bender, E. I. (1976). Self-help groups in Western society: History and prospects. *The Journal of Applied Behavioral Science, 12*(3), 265–282. https://doi.org/10.1177/002188637601200302

Krentzman, A. R. (2021). Helping clients engage with remote mutual aid for addiction recovery during COVID-19 and beyond. *Alcoholism Treatment Quarterly, 39*(3), 348–365. https://doi.org/10.1080/07347324.2021.1917324

Lawn, S., Battersby, M. W., Pols, R. G., Lawrence, J., Parry, T., & Urukalo, M. (2007). The mental health expert patient: Findings from a pilot study of a generic chronic condition self-management programme for people with mental illness. *The International Journal of Social Psychiatry, 53*(1), 63–74. https://doi.org/10.1177/0020764007075010

Lieberman, M. A. (1990). A group therapist perspective on self-help groups. *International Journal of Group Psychotherapy, 40*(3), 251–278. https://doi.org/10.1080/00207284.1990.11490608

Lyons, N., Cooper, C., & Lloyd-Evans, B. (2021). A systematic review and meta-analysis of group peer support interventions for people experiencing mental health conditions. *BMC Psychiatry, 21*(1), Article 315. https://doi.org/10.1186/s12888-021-03321-z

Marino, C. "K.," Child, B., & Campbell Krasinski, V. (2016). Sharing Experience Learned Firsthand (SELF): Self-disclosure of lived experience in mental health services and supports. *Psychiatric Rehabilitation Journal, 39*(2), 154–160. https://doi.org/10.1037/prj0000171

Markowitz, F. E. (2015). Involvement in mental health self-help groups and recovery. *Health Sociology Review, 24*(2), 199–212. https://doi.org/10.1080/14461242.2015.1015149

Mbao, M., Zisman Ilani, Y., Gold, A., Myers, A., Walker, R., & Fortuna, K. L. (2021). Co-production development of a decision support tool for peers and service users to choose technologies to support recovery. *Patient Experience Journal, 8*(3), 45–63. https://doi.org/10.35680/2372-0247.1563

McGovern, W., Addison, M., & McGovern, R. (2022). Negotiating "self-stigma" and an "addicted identity" in traditional 12-step self-help groups. In M. Addison,

W. McGovern, & R. McGovern (Eds.), *Drugs, identity and stigma* (pp. 247–269). Palgrave Macmillan. https://doi.org/10.1007/978-3-030-98286-7_11

McKay, C., Nugent, K. L., Johnsen, M., Eaton, W. W., & Lidz, C. W. (2018). A systematic review of evidence for the clubhouse model of psychosocial rehabilitation. *Administration and Policy in Mental Health and Mental Health Services Research, 45,* 28–47. https://doi.org/10.1007/s10488-016-0760-3

Mercer, F., Miler, J. A., Pauly, B., Carver, H., Hnízdilová, K., Foster, R., & Parkes, T. (2021). Peer support and overdose prevention responses: A systematic "state-of-the-art" review. *International Journal of Environmental Research and Public Health, 18*(22), Article 12073. https://doi.org/10.3390/ijerph182212073

Metz, M., Elfeddali, I., Veerbeek, M., de Beurs, E., Beekman, A., & van der Feltz-Cornelis, C. (2018). Effectiveness of a multi-faceted blended eHealth intervention during intake supporting patients and clinicians in shared decision making: A cluster randomised controlled trial in a specialist mental health outpatient setting. *PLOS ONE, 13*(6), Article e0199795. https://doi.org/10.1371/journal.pone.0199795

Minkowitz, T. (2010). Abolishing mental health laws to comply with the Convention on the Rights of Persons With Disabilities. In B. Sherry & P. Weller (Eds.), *Rethinking rights-based mental health laws* (pp. 151–177). Hart Publishing.

Mullen, J. N., Levitt, A., & Markoulakis, R. (2023). Supporting individuals with mental health and/or addictions issues through patient navigation: A scoping review. *Community Mental Health Journal, 59*(1), 35–56. https://doi.org/10.1007/s10597-022-00982-2

Munson, M. R., Jaccard, J., Scott, L. D., Jr., Moore, K. L., Narendorf, S. C., Cole, A. R., Shimizu, R., Rodwin, A. H., Jenefsky, N., Davis, M., & Gilmer, T. (2021). Outcomes of a metaintervention to improve treatment engagement among young adults with serious mental illnesses: Application of a pilot randomized explanatory design. *Journal of Adolescent Health, 69*(5), 790–796. https://doi.org/10.1016/j.jadohealth.2021.04.023

Myrick, K., & del Vecchio, P. (2016). Peer support services in the behavioral healthcare workforce: State of the field. *Psychiatric Rehabilitation Journal, 39*(3), 197–203. https://doi.org/10.1037/prj0000188

National Association of Peer Supporters. (2013). *National practice guidelines for peer supporters.* https://www.peersupportworks.org/wp-content/uploads/2021/02/nationalguidelines_updated.pdf

Ostrow, L., & Hayes, S. L. (2015). Leadership and characteristics of nonprofit mental health peer-run organizations nationwide. *Psychiatric Services, 66*(4), 421–425. https://doi.org/10.1176/appi.ps.201400080

Ostrow, L., Steinwachs, D., Leaf, P. J., & Naeger, S. (2017). Medicaid reimbursement of mental health peer-run organizations: Results of a national survey. *Administration and Policy in Mental Health and Mental Health Services Research, 44,* 501–511. https://doi.org/10.1007/s10488-015-0675-4

Patient Protection and Affordable Care Act, Pub. L. 111–148, 42 U.S.C. §§ 18001–18121 (2010).

Paudel, S., Sharma, N., Joshi, A., & Randall, M. (2018). Development of a shared decision making model in a community mental health center. *Community Mental Health Journal, 54*(1), 1–6. https://doi.org/10.1007/s10597-017-0134-7

Pfeiffer, P. N., Heisler, M., Piette, J. D., Rogers, M. A., & Valenstein, M. (2011). Efficacy of peer support interventions for depression: A meta-analysis. *General Hospital Psychiatry, 33*(1), 29–36. https://doi.org/10.1016/j.genhosppsych.2010. 10.002

Pistrang, N., Barker, C., & Humphreys, K. (2008). Mutual help groups for mental health problems: A review of effectiveness studies. *American Journal of Community Psychology, 42*(1–2), 110–121. https://doi.org/10.1007/s10464-008-9181-0

Repper, J., & Carter, T. (2011). A review of the literature on peer support in mental health services. *Journal of Mental Health, 20*(4), 392–411. https://doi.org/10.3109/ 09638237.2011.583947

Rüsch, N., & Kösters, M. (2021). Honest, Open, Proud to support disclosure decisions and to decrease stigma's impact among people with mental illness: Conceptual review and meta-analysis of program efficacy. *Social Psychiatry and Psychiatric Epidemiology, 56*(9), 1513–1526. https://doi.org/10.1007/s00127-021-02076-y

Schladitz, K., Weitzel, E. C., Löbner, M., Soltmann, B., Jessen, F., Pfennig, A., Riedel-Heller, S. G., & Gühne, U. (2023). Experiencing (shared) decision making: Results from a qualitative study of people with mental illness and their family members. *Healthcare, 11*(16), Article 2237. https://doi.org/10.3390/healthcare11162237

Schuster, J.-P., Hoertel, N., & Limosin, F. (2011). The man behind Philippe Pinel: Jean-Baptiste Pussin (1746–1811). *The British Journal of Psychiatry, 198*(3), Article 241. https://doi.org/10.1192/bjp.198.3.241a

Simmons, M. B., Coates, D., Batchelor, S., Dimopoulos-Bick, T., & Howe, D. (2018). The CHOICE pilot project: Challenges of implementing a combined peer work and shared decision-making programme in an early intervention service. *Early Intervention in Psychiatry, 12*(5), 964–971. https://doi.org/10.1111/eip.12527

Simmons, M. B., & Gooding, P. M. (2017). Spot the difference: Shared decision-making and supported decision-making in mental health. *Irish Journal of Psychological Medicine, 34*(4), 275–286. https://doi.org/10.1017/ipm.2017.59

Smit, D., Miguel, C., Vrijsen, J. N., Groeneweg, B., Spijker, J., & Cuijpers, P. (2022). The effectiveness of peer support for individuals with mental illness: Systematic review and meta-analysis. *Psychological Medicine, 53*(11), 5332–5341. https:// doi.org/10.1017/S0033291722002422

Swarbrick, M. (2011). Self-help and peer-operated services. In A. Rudnick & D. Roe (Eds.), *Serious mental illness: Person-centered approaches* (pp. 301–312). Radcliffe Publishing.

Swarbrick, M., Gill, K. J., & Pratt, C. W. (2016). Impact of peer delivered wellness coaching. *Psychiatric Rehabilitation Journal, 39*(3), 234–238. https://psycnet.apa. org/doi/10.1037/prj0000187

Thomas, E. C., Simmons, M. B., Mathai, C., & Salzer, M. S. (2023). Peer-facilitated decision making in mental health: Promises, pitfalls, and recommendations for research and practice. *Psychiatric Services, 74*(4), 401–406. https://doi.org/10.1176/ appi.ps.20220086

Tracy, K., & Wallace, S. P. (2016). Benefits of peer support groups in the treatment of addiction. *Substance Abuse and Rehabilitation, 7*, 143–154. https://doi.org/ 10.2147/SAR.S81535

Van Tosh, L., Ralph, R. O., & Campbell, J. (2000). The rise of consumerism. *Psychiatric Rehabilitation Skills, 4*(3), 383–409. https://doi.org/10.1080/10973430008408630

Videka, L., Neale, J., Page, C., Buche, J., Beck, A. J., Wayment, C., & Gaiser, M. (2019). *National analysis of peer support providers: Practice settings, requirements, roles, and reimbursement*. Behavioral Health Workforce.

Voss, M., Barrett, T. S., Lapidos, A., Werner, P., Bennett, P., Campbell, A., & Van Komen, A. (2022). *Peer support workforce survey: Professional activities, skills, job satisfaction, and financial well-being*. SSRN. https://papers.ssrn.com/sol3/papers.cfm?abstract_id=4273593

White, S., Foster, R., Marks, J., Morshead, R., Goldsmith, L., Barlow, S., Sin, J., & Gillard, S. (2020). The effectiveness of one-to-one peer support in mental health services: A systematic review and meta-analysis. *BMC Psychiatry, 20*, Article 534. https://doi.org/10.1186/s12888-020-02923-3

World Health Organization. (2019). *One-to-one peer support by and for people with lived experience: WHO QualityRights guidance module*. https://iris.who.int/bitstream/handle/10665/329591/9789241516785-eng.pdf

Wu, J. R., Iwanaga, K., Chan, F., Lee, B., Chen, X., Walker, R., Fortuna, K. L., & Brooks, J. M. (2023). Positive organizational psychology factors as serial multiple mediators of the relationship between organization support and job satisfaction among peer support specialists. *Journal of Occupational Rehabilitation, 33*(1), 121–133. https://doi.org/10.1007/s10926-022-10054-7

Yamaguchi, S., Taneda, A., Matsunaga, A., Sasaki, N., Mizuno, M., Sawada, Y., Sakata, M., Fukui, S., Hisanaga, F., Bernick, P., & Ito, J. (2017). Efficacy of a peer-led, recovery-oriented shared decision-making system: A pilot randomized controlled trial. *Psychiatric Services, 68*(12), 1307–1311. https://doi.org/10.1176/appi.ps.201600544

Zisman-Ilani, Y., & Byrne, L. (2023). Shared decision making and peer support: New directions for research and practice. *Psychiatric Services, 74*(4), 427–428. https://doi.org/10.1176/appi.ps.20220407

Zisman-Ilani, Y., Hayes, D., & Fancourt, D. (2023). Promoting social prescribing in psychiatry—Using shared decision-making and peer support. *JAMA Psychiatry, 80*(8), 759–760. https://doi.org/10.1001/jamapsychiatry.2023.0788

6

PRACTICAL GUIDE TO SHARED DECISION MAKING FOR MENTAL HEALTH

PATRICK W. CORRIGAN AND VARDHA KHARBANDA

This chapter is specifically written for the shared decision making (SDM) user: for the service provider who works with people who are making decisions about health, wellness, or psychosocial goals; for these people themselves; and perhaps for other stakeholders in the process. We have synthesized recommendations, guidelines, and tools to form a step-by-step guide.

The chapter begins with a review of multiple consensus documents representing practice guidelines that are the basis for the recommendations herein. In addition to briefly describing methods used to form guidelines, we provide online links to guidelines, where the reader can review more details about the recommendations. Next, we review the goals that underlie SDM. The conceptual underpinnings of goals in this chapter were unpacked throughout the earlier chapters in this book. The assignment here is to frame goals in terms of actual practice: Why might a person engage service providers to make decisions about life goals? Because of this focus, Chapter 6 is light on citations. Next, we describe roles relevant to SDM—that is, the person pursuing life goal(s), or PPLG;[1] service provider; and other stakeholder—and

---

[1]We admit that PPLG is a clunky acronym. We picked it to stress the central reason why people with lived experience engage in SDM: because they choose to pursue a personally-identified life goal.

https://doi.org/10.1037/0000478-006
Shared Decision Making and Serious Mental Illness, P. W. Corrigan (Editor)

corresponding logistics. We then summarize the heart of this chapter: the seven steps that make up SDM. These steps are detailed as tools with corresponding worksheets that facilitate SDM.

CONSENSUS GUIDELINES

Consensus guidelines are a comprehensive list of provider actions that assist people in health, wellness, and psychosocial goals; the focus of this chapter is consensus guidelines for SDM. Consensus guidelines have several benefits. They typically represent an evidence-based attempt to understand and affect a person's life; they are cookbooks, as it were, which providers readily pick up and use to realize the focal procedure (e.g., SDM). These cookbooks then form the basis of training and subsequent supervision. They are also used for fidelity checks: Is the provider doing the practice as outlined in the guidelines? This kind of cookbook is also the catalyst for ongoing development and implementation. Stakeholders can provide feedback for subsequent evolution as providers implement guidelines.

A systematic synthesis of 10 peer-reviewed papers outlined several principles for the creation of consensus guidelines on specific health conditions that are organized into six areas (El-Harakeh et al., 2019):

1. Disease-related factors, which are described in terms of health and economic burden as well as equity relevance and urgency.

2. Interest, which refers to priorities by stakeholders (e.g., service consumers, health professionals, other stakeholders).

3. Practice, that is, the relevance as facilitators or barriers to best practice.

4. Guideline development, which involves the potential for enhancing current guidelines as well as replacing poor frameworks.

5. Intervention impact, which refers to the effects on health outcomes, economics, health care systems, and health equity.

6. Implementation considerations, which involve existing information about feasibility, fidelity, and resources that support dissemination and implementation.

Building guidelines often begins with a subcommittee of professional or advocacy groups that use these principles to address an agreed on focal health practice. Consensus guidelines have emerged as a large force in health care practice with different professions tackling such guidelines for almost every major health condition. Development of consensus guidelines begins with a careful and comprehensive review of the existing research literature summarizing studies on the focal service (i.e., SDM) with special value given to research that has identified and tested key ingredients in the treatment.

The Cochrane Library is a major source of these reviews (see https://www.cochranelibrary.com). Additional research unpacks these ingredients in terms of discrete steps (e.g., for SDM, making sense of one's values, translating decisions into action plans). The review includes a clear statement of the goal of the intervention (e.g., to assist people to make decisions that lead to actions about specific health needs and life goals) that serves as the anchor for discerning steps to include or that might be extraneous.

Consensus panels then sift through the information and agree not only on common definitions for problems, goals, and corresponding interventions but also get some sense of the steps in which these definitions can be rolled out. This is an iterative process that includes in-the-field tests of all elements of the guideline.

Who might compose consensus panels? The panels are often dominated by professional groups and guilds that reflect the interests of specific providers, such as physicians, nurses, and other allied health professions. This kind of guild-based approach has value because interested members come together based on similar sets of learning materials and experiences. In the process, they create guidelines (like the consensus guidelines mentioned later in the chapter) that reflect their insights into barriers and facilitators of specific goals. However, these guild-based approaches also have their limits. They might yield guidelines that favor their profession over another—for example, by asserting that psychiatrists have sole authority over diagnosis. In addition, these guild-based consensus panels often exclude perspectives of other stakeholders, including people with lived experience and their networks such as family, friends, and faith-based communities. The rise of the Patient-Centered Outcomes Research Institute (see https://www.pcori.org) has led to consensus reviews through a systematic partnership of all stakeholders. The recovery-based health care system is especially notable in that it includes people with lived experience in the development of principles, practices, services, and interventions that support recovery.

Table 6.1 provides a list of SDM consensus guidelines developed in the United States and around the world. Although one set of guidelines is specific to pediatrics, the majority are more generic to health conditions in general. The Substance Abuse and Mental Health Services Administration (SAMHSA)

TABLE 6.1. Existing Consensus Guidelines for Shared Decision Making

Group or organization	Title of guidelines
Organizations in the United States of America	
Agency for Healthcare Research and Quality (2017)	The CAHPS Ambulatory Care Improvement Guide: Practical Strategies for Improving Patient Experience
American Academy of Pediatrics (Opel, 2018)	A 4-Step Framework for Shared Decision-Making in Pediatrics
Foundation for Health Care Quality (Dr. Robert Bree Collaborative, 2019)	Shared Decision Making
National Quality Forum (2017)	Shared Decision Making: A Standard of Care for All Patients
Substance Abuse and Mental Health Services Administration (2011, 2016)	Supporting Choice: Helping Others Make Important Decisions
	Decisions in Recovery: Treatment for Opioid Use Disorder
U.S. Preventive Services Task Force (2022)	Collaboration and Shared Decision-Making Between Patients and Clinicians in Preventive Health Care Decisions and US Preventive Services Task Force Recommendations
International organizations	
EBSCO (Elwyn & Durand, 2018)	Mastering Shared Decision Making: The When, Why, and How
General Medical Council (2020)	Decision-Making and Consent
Scottish Government (2019)	Shared Decision-Making in Realistic Medicine: What Works
National Health Service England (2019)	Shared Decision Making: Summary Guide
National Institute for Health and Care Excellence (NICE; 2021)	Shared Decision Making: NICE Guideline
Shared Decision Making Collaborative (2015)	A Consensus Statement

has two sets of SDM guidelines related to behavioral health. The first is specific to antipsychotic medications and includes such issues as comparing available antipsychotic drugs and their key side effects; finding information about other treatments, service options, and complementary approaches; considering preferences on the role of antipsychotic medications in one's recovery plan; and creating a personalized summary to share with one's service provider (SAMHSA, 2011). The second set of guidelines is related to medication-assisted treatments for opioid use disorder (SAMHSA, 2016).

ACTIVATE PARTIES IN SHARED DECISION MAKING AND THEIR GOALS

In general, many of these health service guidelines come from the physical health care system and hence represent the presumed link between illness (summarized as diagnosis) and corresponding evidenced-based treatments. SDM is a bit of a different process when also applied more broadly to life goals related to psychosocial functions: education, employment, independent living, and relationships. As can be seen in Figure 6.1, we frame SDM in terms of three groups of actors: (a) the person receiving services to meet life goals, (b) those providing SDM, and (c) other interested stakeholders. We provide a thorough description of each group as a way to situate SDM in a helping enterprise. Table 6.2 summarizes the key roles of these three groups.

Person Pursuing Life Goal(s)

SDM is rooted in the priorities and actions of the PPLG. As such, it reflects the first principles of person-centered care and self-determination theory. The PPLG's goals are often based on mental illness, which evokes ideas of symptoms and dysfunction that are important targets of psychiatric services. People want to diminish anxiety and depression or enhance ways to think clearly despite ongoing stress. Life goals, however, reflect a broader horizon beyond health and wellness that represent the same broad spectrum of aspirations that are pursued by every adult, including education, meaning, employment, career, income, independent living, relationships, and spiritual life. SDM is grounded by the person's description of their goals, be they health and wellness or psychosocial. One of the first tasks of SDM is to help people give voice to those goals.

FIGURE 6.1. Key Actors in Shared Decision Making

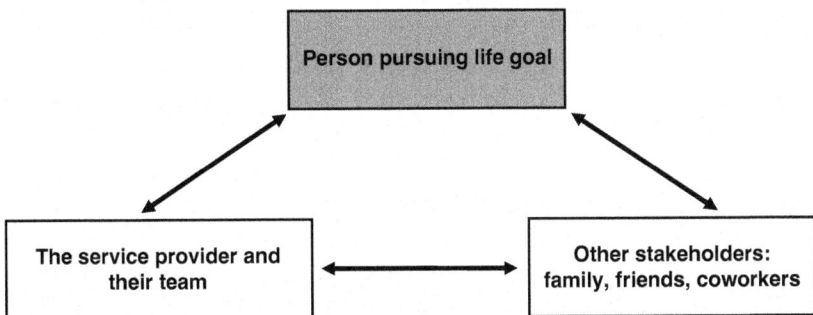

TABLE 6.2. Tasks for Groups That Might Participate in Shared Decision Making

Participant and definition	Task
PPLG: Individual who is the central focus of the SDM process; this may be defined as a partnership (e.g., spouses, polyamorous relationships, or otherwise committed couples)	Defines the purpose of SDM Sets agenda Has final decision-making authority
Service provider: Although services are provided by a team, one member of that team may assume responsibility for coordinating the SDM process; we call them the provider doing SDM	Facilitates SDM Provides some "expertise" in terms of goal area
Other stakeholders: Family, friends, and others who may have a perspective or role in the SDM process and goals—if the PPLG chooses to involve them	Offer the benefit of their perspectives to people with life goal(s), who are the focus of SDM and might add these perspectives to the SDM process; the person per se has final authority regarding who is included and how; family-centered decision making (described later in this chapter) offers an additional perspective of SDM, especially in terms of participating family members

Note. PPLG = person pursuing life goal(s); SDM = shared decision making.

A Single PPLG

Goals are dynamic: A person's perspectives often change over time as they become better aware of diverse parameters that influence goals. Dynamics are partly driven by comprehension (i.e., increased understanding of evidence about a goal and strategies to accomplish it) and partly by reprioritization (i.e., aspirations for a specific goal or component of a goal evolve with greater knowledge). For example, the goal of completing an educational program to pursue a specific career may diminish when the person realizes the time demands of corresponding programs. Hence, the PPLG and provider need to avoid casting single static goals as the sole focus of SDM.

Multiple goals may often be the focus of SDM. Take, for example, Louise Bird, a PPLG who wants to pursue education and work and finish a certificate program in accounting to obtain a business career in finance. These goals are not usually independent. For example, Louise's education and work goals might be closely linked: Earning a professional certification is primary to pursuing a job in related fields. Hence, these dual goals might yield a single SDM process and plan. Separately, Louise may see decisions about home and housing to be fairly independent of where she works. The SDM process here might be separate. As always, making decisions about goals and independence is a dynamic process driven by the PPLG, so individual sets of SDM plans and actions vary in terms of their interconnectedness.

Beyond a Single PPLG

In some situations, the focus of SDM may be led by multiple people instead of one PPLG, most notably, situations in which life partners (e.g., spouses) have a shared goal—for instance: "Should we move across the country for new jobs?" Implicit in the goal and corresponding SDM are the linked interests of the partner that represent a spoken sense of commitment. As partners, the two focal people have equal authority over goals and are responsible for participating in the process of achieving these goals. Hence, both parties are fully engaged in SDM.

Partnered relationships typically do not include extended families—for example, PPLG and parents, siblings, or the broader clan—at least in Western cultures. The difference here lies in the absence of shared goals. True, a PPLG living with their parents has goals of interest to the broader family. However, the goal is owned by the PPLG. As discussed later in the chapter in the section on family-centered decision making, the PPLG might decide to include other stakeholders for added perspective and assistance in an action plan, but the PPLG typically has the final decision. That does not mean that the parents in this example have no goals of their own, but their SDM process is a separate one owned by the parents: How do we make homelife more conducive to our adult child with mental illness? The parents become separate people pursuing life goal(s)—that is, PPLGs—and the child with mental illness may be a stakeholder in their SDM. Note that SDM focusing on PPLG goals is an independent process from that focusing on parent goals.

PPLGs may select other stakeholders that might help in SDM. This might include educators when pursuing academic goals, supervisors or coworkers relevant to career goals, and faith-based leaders for spiritual priorities. The role of these stakeholders is a bit circumscribed with a special focus on additional perspectives that might inform the goal, solutions to the goal, or implementation of the action plan.

Service Provider

Services for the PPLG are often provided by a team. SDM is a partnership between the PPLG and a service provider who has dedicated responsibility for this kind of decision-making process; we call them the provider doing

SDM (P-SDM).[2] By "dedicated," we mean a professional or paraprofessional who has agreed to take on SDM roles and partner with the person to advance their goals. Services providers have two broad foci in this partnership: to (a) facilitate an open discussion between the PPLG and provider about goals driving this discussion and (b) use their expertise to educate the PPLG about the goal ("What is it?") and strategies to facilitate it ("What might I do with it?").

SDM as it developed in physical health care framed service providers as experts. These experts were typically physicians (both primary and specialty care); nurse practitioners or physician assistants; or providers from allied health professions, such as nutritionists, physical therapists, podiatrists, or mental health counselors. Expertise here reflects the assumption of a one-to-one correspondence between a diagnosed health condition or wellness focus and corresponding evidence-based treatments. The expert service provider is expected to have a broad knowledge of diagnosis and treatments, which is shared with PPLGs to inform their decision making. Service providers, though, do not decide what is the best way to obtain goals based on their expert knowledge. Rather, they provide a menu of options with clear descriptions; this includes a willingness to more fully expand on descriptions (including online or paper resources) or seek additional consultation for other relevant service providers as requested by the PPLG.

When asked, the P-SDM might also review research on the relative effects of specific interventions. Hence, P-SDMs as experts may be an authoritative resource of options from which the person might select treatment. Authoritative does not mean exclusive, however; the provider needs to be willing to explore complementary or other nontraditional approaches to goals should PPLGs express interest. P-SDMs need to be mindful of information overload. More facts about an intervention are not necessarily better if the PPLG becomes overwhelmed with possibilities. Like much of SDM, sharing knowledge is a dynamic process; greater knowledge is shared when the PPLG seeks clarity.

The role of expertise is less clear for SDM embedded in rehabilitation and recovery approaches that focus on goals related to, for example, education, career, independent living, or relationships. Consider work-related goals as an example: issues related to career, employment, and income. The one-to-one correspondence that defines expertise in much of physical health care is less definitive in work goals. Vocational counselors do not diagnose a client

---

[2]Another awkward acronym to be sure, but once again, we wish to fully name the provider side of this dyad: the P-SDM.

with "failure-to-work" based on key indicators; there is nothing in the fifth edition, text revision, of the *Diagnostic and Statistical Manual of Mental Disorders* (*DSM-5-TR*; American Psychiatric Association, 2022) that provides this kind of direction. Hence, there is not a black-and-white set of tools that suggests what specifically PPLGs might do with the service provider to achieve work goals. The provider's expertise in this case seems to be in the process of SDM exploration. What might the service provider do to help PPLGs better identify elements of their goals and actions that might resolve them? Many exemplary recovery-based programs, such as Individual Placement and Support, supported education, and assertive community treatment, have already integrated goal exploration and SDM as central processes in their programs.

SDM may be best facilitated by a single service provider: the P-SDM, who works with the PPLG throughout the process. Service providers of all backgrounds might serve as P-SDMs, including physicians, nurse practitioners, social workers, nutritionists, and physical therapists; however, people who are care coordinators, providers, or job coaches are often best positioned to do this. Individual providers should consider two factors when becoming P-SDMs:

1. Time and place: The service provider must have sufficient time and a private place to meet with the PPLG and unpack the elements of SDM. Frequently, health care providers with other service demands (e.g., busy clinics with stacked-up appointments) are not able to do justice to SDM.

2. Problem-solving interrelatedness skills: These are the communication skills that facilitate SDM. Service providers with some sort of counseling skills might find SDM roles easier, although P-SDMs need not be formally certified counselors. Many health care professionals master communication skills as central to their practice.

Other Stakeholders

Goals and SDM occur in a social world; they typically involve the PPLG's family or their broader social network, including community and faith-based leaders. Work-related goals, for example, might involve employers, supervisors, and coworkers. Education goals could include instructors, school administrators, and other students. Each of these parties may have perspectives that enlighten goals as well as serve adjunct roles in implementing SDM plans. However, the PPLG typically has the ultimate decision over who is included in SDM as well as how that group might change during the SDM process.

SEVEN STEPS OF SHARED DECISION MAKING

Table 6.3 summarizes the seven steps of SDM along with key actions and outcomes. Sometimes, single steps can be extracted alone as a tool to advance any snags in the existing SDM process. For example, Step 5—consideration of the pros and cons of a specific action—might help the SDM dyad understand the specifics of the intervention and adaptations that better fit the PPLG's perspectives.[3]

Step 1: Engage the Person in Decision Making

SDM begins with a brief overview by summarizing its seven steps for the PPLG (see Table 6.3)—just a brief introduction so the PPLG has some sense of where the process will go. SDM rests on the PPLG's assumption that this process will somehow be beneficial and that SDM, in conjunction with the PPLG's skills and attitudes, will eventually lead to some change. PPLGs who have been unsuccessful in such ventures in the past may approach SDM half-heartedly, having little confidence in its value. Hence, the first job on Worksheet 1 is for the PPLG to complete a 10-point scale ranging from 1 (*not confident*) to 10 (*extremely confident*) answering the question, "How confident do you feel in your ability to achieve your goals?" The P-SDM then initiates a discussion of the PPLG's responses.

Do not disregard low scores but, instead, empathize with them and invite a discussion of hesitations. To accomplish Step 1 and engage the PPLG in the process of SDM, use the basic questions of information gathering: why, who, when, where, and what.

Why?

The goal of SDM is to help PPLGs identify key goals and then corresponding actions that help people accomplish them. Why exactly is the PPLG joining with the service provider to set goals and make action plans? This might seem to be an obvious question for the P-SDM but can sometimes be disorienting for the PPLG. They may not realize that goal setting and action plans are separate experiences from the overall service. The answer to the why question is joint recognition by PPLG and P-SDM that an understanding of personal goals, varied ways to address goals, and subsequent personally

---

[3]The worksheets that the P-SDM and PPLG complete jointly to implement corresponding tasks are available online (see the Resources tab at https://www.apa.org/pubs/books/shared-decision-making-serious-mental-illness).

TABLE 6.3. Seven Steps of Shared Decision Making

Step	Actions and outcomes

1. Engage the person in decision making:
  - Launch a helping relationship.
  - Conduct an orientation and provide education about the process.
  - Develop a decision-making perspective.
  - Review the person's sense of self-efficacy.
	Review the role of perceived self-efficacy in goal attainment. Assess the person's optimism about SDM. This is done in a counseling relationship in which the PPLG feels free to explore goals and actions.

2. Identify goals, especially in terms of personal values.	Identify goals that are specific, measurable, actionable, realistic, and timely. Consider multiple goals and their independence. Be mindful of information overload and the efficiency trade-off.
3. Share expert information about goals, corresponding actions, and composite tasks: Discuss care providers' expertise about goals and ways to accomplish them.	The care provider summarizes the state of the evidence about understanding specific goals, barriers to goals, and strategies that help a person achieve them.
4. Specify a broad list of actions to achieve goals.	The person and care provider make a preliminary list of actions that will help a person attain the goal.
5. Weigh the pros and cons of each option.	Weigh the pros and cons of each option in terms of meeting goals as well as any unintended effects. *See Worksheet 4* (see the Resources tab at https://www.apa.org/pubs/books/shared-decision-making-serious-mental-illness).
6. Make a comprehensive action plan.	Specify what actions will be done on a timeline with place and other people included as appropriate. Specify outcomes that can be used to evaluate the success of the plan. *See Worksheet 5* (see the Resources tab at https://www.apa.org/pubs/books/shared-decision-making-serious-mental-illness).
7. Evaluate the action plan and revise it when necessary.	Circle back, review the plan, and reconsider actions in terms of success evaluation. Replace or revise actions for better success where appropriate. *See Worksheet 6* (see the Resources tab at https://www.apa.org/pubs/books/shared-decision-making-serious-mental-illness).

Note. SDM = shared decision making; PPLG = person pursing life goal(s).

meaningful actions is a necessary step in addressing what brings the person for service. The P-SDM may briefly orient the PPLG to preparations and steps that compose SDM. Once again, the message is one of flexibility ("We use these strategies to help you move forward.") rather than one etched in stone.

In Worksheet 1, PPLGs write down the health/wellness or psychosocial goal that is the focus of SDM. Remember: SDM largely evolved out of medical practice with a focus on physical and mental health challenges; hence, the person might list a specific illness: recurring major depression or a specific cluster of symptoms and experiences that concern them, such as frequent crying, anhedonia, suicidal ideation, and low energy. SDM, however, has evolved to address the broader life goals common to psychiatric rehabilitation and recovery-based services, including education, work and career, independent living, and meaningful relationships. These are broad topics; people might benefit from discussing with the provider what this means for them.

In addition to the PPLG's specific goal, the "Why?" section of Worksheet 1 asks, "Why will SDM help you [the PPLG] with this condition or personal goal?" Answers to the question might be advanced by the expertise of the P-SDM. In cases, for example, in which SDM occurs during an office visit with a psychiatrist, the provider could inform the person about the facts of major depression: What causes it, what are its symptoms, and how might it be treated. Alternatively, the PPLG can partner with a job coach to unpack and then address barriers to a career. The PPLG and P-SDM may drill down into these questions in Step 3: Share expert information about goals, corresponding actions, and composite tasks. Hence, an iterative approach might help here: moving back and forth between the person's goals and the related condition so PPLGs can better understand their goals.

Who?

Who is involved in the SDM process? The central focus is around the PPLG and service provider dyad. Although the SDM provider facilitates SDM as outlined next, SDM providers need to also explain their role within the larger context of the provider's team. This includes the dyad defining communication processes between PPLG and the broader team. Will the SDM provider contact the broader team with action plans as they develop, or does the PPLG want to do this? In addition, the PPLG and provider dyad should decide whether additional stakeholders—for example, family, friends, or coworkers—might be included in SDM. This decision is facilitated by reviewing the costs and benefits of other stakeholder perspectives in understanding goals as well as their possible role in subsequently implementing the action plan. As stated throughout this book, other stakeholders are identified only by the PPLG. The PPLG determines the extent of other stakeholder roles and when or where they might participate. However, other stakeholders may decide not to accept these conditions and back out of SDM.

As outlined earlier, the PPLG might be two people in partnered relationships with clearly shared goals. In this case, the SDM provider should review the two partners' expectations about both parties fully participating in the seven steps of SDM and corresponding worksheets.

When?

SDM does not need to be a set time or separate service sessions but, rather, maybe incorporated into the broader provision of interventions. Typical is the interaction in which the P-SDM has summarized the person's concerns (e.g., how to get a satisfying career) followed by a description of possible ways to address the concern (e.g., supported employment with a job coach). As always, this decision best emerges through the SDM dyad. Generally, though, the more formal process outlined herein may be indicated when action plans in response to goals have failed to be designed or have not been effective after being implemented.

"When?" in Worksheet 1 is a simple question. Do PPLGs want to set up extra times to meet with the P-SDM or to do it in the course of normal professional interactions? Is SDM going to be a one-time experience, perhaps arising extemporaneously in the context of a specific service moment—for example, with the job coach? Or, after learning more about SDM, might the PPLG decide subsequent meetings service would be beneficial? If so, does the PPLG want to schedule regular times to meet (date and times) or do it as the opportunity arises?

Where?

The dyad engaged in SDM also needs a place to work. Although exam rooms in clinics are one place to do this, the dyad might want to review goals related to on-the-job stress before entering work for the day. This could be done in the provider's car or across the table at a coffee shop. Regardless of specifics, the "place" must be sufficiently private and quiet so the dyad can work without distraction. Providers also need to make sure they have sufficient time to talk and will not be interrupted by the next appointment.

What?

SDM comprises seven steps (see Table 6.3). We reiterate that the PPLG and provider dyad may decide to alter steps in the moment to address the current exigencies of SDM. We illustrate each step by focusing on one case example (see Exhibit 6.1).

Step 2: Identify Goals, Especially in Terms of Personal Values

Step 2 helps PPLGs to make sense of the goals driving their SDM; look at Worksheet 2. In some ways, worksheet specifics parallel the who, when, where, and what of Worksheet 1 on preparing for SDM. The worksheet begins by transferring the personal goals identified in Step 1 and Worksheet 1. Often, the PPLG does not have a complete understanding of what is involved in specific goals. This may take the kind of expert information shared in Step 3. Hence, Steps 2 and 3 may be iterative processes in which PPLGs provide a preliminary sense of goal, learn more about the related life domain, and then return to better describe their aspirations.

PPLGs and P-SDM address the "what" of goal identification: "What does the person want to achieve through this goal?" This step, like SDM overall, is driven by personal values—what the PPLG wants to fill out a satisfying life. Hence, the P-SDM's goal is to be supportive. Reflective listening is especially important here. People benefit from hearing how others perceive their preferences as a way to more fully develop them. The PPLG is asked to further develop the idea in detail. The "what" question includes describing how achievement will be measured. This is less an evaluation question (although Step 5 returns to evaluating benefits and limitations of the decisions) and more to avail benefits of careful definition; namely, what exactly does the

EXHIBIT 6.1. Case Example: Fong Tsang

Fong Tsang is a 35-year-old man of Chinese descent wondering whether he should go to a local community college to earn a technical certificate. Figure 6.2 is the completed version of Worksheet 1 for Fong Tsang. He was unsure about his ability to achieve goals, reporting only a 4. As a result, the provider who was doing shared decision making (SDM), Leticia Porter, engaged him in a discussion about previous efforts during which he sought to achieve goals, focusing on possible successes. This exchange led Fong to be a bit more hopeful, raising his score to a 6.

When Leticia and Fong first met, Fong said his goal was to get some kind of "professional certificate" to make himself more employable. Specifically, he wanted SDM to better define the steps he needed to pursue and achieve to enroll and participate in a certificate program. He named his mother Li as a supportive stakeholder. Moreover, Fong had a deep relationship with the local Chinese Christian Union Church, where he met with Reverend Lam for regular guidance. Fong thought SDM meetings would need to be regularly scheduled and wanted to have these meetings at the local community college, Olive-Harvey College, where he might pursue the certificate.

Note. Case examples in this book are hypothetical.

FIGURE 6.2. Fong's Preparing for Shared Decision Making

Worksheet 1
Preparing for Shared Decision Making (SDM)

How confident do you feel in your ability to achieve your goals? On a scale of 1 to 10, rate your perceived self-efficacy.

[Scale: Not at all (1) to Very Much (10), with 4 circled]

WHY?

Name the health condition(s) or personal goal(s) for which you would like to do SDM.
Pursuing a professional certificate

Why will SDM help you with the condition or personal goal?
Define the steps to get into school and be successful

WHO?

What is your name?: Fong Tsang	What is your service: provider's name? Leticia Porter

Other Stakeholders (These may be modified as SDM progresses)

1. Li Tsang (Mother)	2. Reverend Lam (Minister)
3.	4.

WHEN?

• I would like it to be <u>part of the regularly scheduled service:</u>	✓ • I would like it to be <u>specifically scheduled</u> • Specific Date: 1/15/23 & Time: 9:30 AM AM/PM

WHERE?

I would like the SDM sessions to be conducted in...

• Exam rooms in clinics	• At home	• In a community center
• Office or consultation room	• Over a video call	• During a walk or other leisure activity

✓ • Other (Please specify): At the Olive-Harvey City College

WHAT?

These are the 7 steps of SDM (Engage, Identify Goals, Share Expertise, Specify Actions, Weigh Options, Plan, Evaluate & Revise)

PPLG do to achieve the goal? This leads to specifying actions that the PPLG might pursue. Specifying actions is key to Step 6 in which the action plan is drafted. Worksheet 2 provides the first opportunity for PPLGs to brainstorm possible actions.

It is helpful to designate a P-SDM facilitator so they can work with the overall team to meet the various elements of the action plan. In dealing with finding and keeping a job, for example, the team decides who will act as job coach, tracking all the activities related to hiring and maintaining a job. Outlining these roles illustrates the mutuality of the SDM process. The PPLG creates a plan specifying actions therein. However, the P-SDM and provider team assume responsibility for specific elements of the plan as they occur.

The personalized professional learning goals and personalized shared decision making teams need to clearly determine where and when actions should take place to achieve specific goals. For example:

- Where: Education-related goals might be best addressed on campus, whereas work-related goals are better suited to the workplace.

- When: Actions can be scheduled within a specific time range (e.g., meeting a faculty advisor during office hours from 12 p.m. to 2 p.m.) or left flexible based on availability (e.g., meeting a supervisor during regular work hours: 9 a.m. to 5 p.m.).

The goal is to ensure clarity and feasibility in planning so everyone involved knows exactly how and when to act. This approach balances structure with flexibility depending on the context of the task.

Example

In Figure 6.3, Fong states on Worksheet 2 that his psychosocial goal is to get a professional certificate. He admits uncertainty about the field and prerequisites for enrollment. As he develops his thoughts, Fong realizes his ongoing struggles with mental health challenges may undermine the pursuit of this certificate and hence hopes SDM can suggest some action therein. Leticia Porter is a student support center professional at Olive-Harvey College, where Fong wants to pursue the certificate. Services will be provided when the student support office is open or when classes are active at the college.

Step 3: Share Expert Information About Goals, Corresponding Actions, and Composite Tasks

Central to SDM is a fact-finding mission: helping PPLGs to obtain information to enhance decision making. P-SDMs who are members of the service team are a key source of this information; they tend to come from the health or psychosocial service sector in which the decision is anchored. SDM is rooted in existing bodies of knowledge that are useful in understanding life goals and facilitating their accomplishments. Who qualifies to be an expert? Some licenses and certifications indicate an individual has mastered a base of knowledge and practice to define a scope of practice. P-SDMs use this base to share an organized summary of what research says about the targeted psychosocial goal (How do I get a college certificate?). P-SDMs then summarize the variety of treatment options that research has identified as effective for these problems and goals.

FIGURE 6.3. Fong's Goal Identification

Worksheet 2
Identifying Goals In Terms of Personal Values

From Worksheet 1: what is the health condition or psychosocial goal?

Get a professional certificate to get a better job

Let's discuss the health condition or psychosocial goal in detail

Find an appropriate certificate program. Concerned about mental health symptoms as a barrier

What specific outcome or improvement are you hoping for?

Get the certificate

Get help finding a job

How will we measure your goals?

Certificate

Job

What actions might you take to achieve these goals?
Note: Step 3 will provide possible actions

Enroll

Get mental health support

Who is the service provider (s) especially important to the goal: <u>Leticia Porter</u>

Where will the service be provided? <u>Student support center at Olive Harvey</u>

When will the service be provided? <u>When school is in session.</u>

Example

Fong works with Leticia Porter to gather expert information about his goal. Leticia provides Fong with details about the available certificate programs, their prerequisites, and application deadlines. She also informs him about resources like financial aid options, tutoring services, and mental health support available on campus.

During their discussion, Fong shares that he feels overwhelmed by the number of steps involved in enrolling and worries about managing his mental health challenges alongside his studies. Leticia explains how he can break down the process into manageable tasks, such as attending an orientation session, meeting with an academic advisor, and submitting required documents step by step. She also connects him with a counselor who specializes in supporting students with mental health concerns.

Through this process, Fong gains clarity about what pursuing the certificate entails and feels more confident about taking the next steps. Leticia ensures that their meetings occur during her office hours or when Fong is already on campus for other activities, making it convenient for him to access support.

Summary Trees for Psychosocial Goals
Summary trees are concise, visual tools designed to help individuals and providers collaboratively navigate psychosocial goals within the framework of SDM. These tools simplify complex processes by breaking them into actionable steps, ensuring that individuals, referred to as a personalized professionals learning goals, can make informed decisions without being overwhelmed by excessive information. Summary trees emphasize flexibility and personalization, focusing on goals like education, employment, independent living, and meaningful relationships rather than narrowly defined diagnoses. They help anchor the SDM process in practical actions while remaining adaptable to individual needs and values.

The SDM process begins by engaging the individual through a structured but empathetic approach. This involves assessing confidence levels, clarifying personal goals, and understanding why SDM can be beneficial for achieving these objectives. For example, a person aiming to return to school may use a summary tree to outline steps, such as identifying educational programs, integrating mental health support with academic planning, and scheduling regular follow-ups with a provider. These tools ensure that the process remains centered on the individual's values and aspirations while fostering collaboration between the individual and the provider.

Program manuals from organizations like SAMHSA complement summary trees by offering evidence-based strategies for achieving psychosocial goals. Some of these are summarized in Table 6.4 and include aspirations related to employment, independent living, and integrated health care. These manuals are especially strong on the Stage 2 arm of SDM by carefully and comprehensively summarizing the actions necessary to achieve the focal goals.

The bottom half of the list in Table 6.4 reflects goals more consistent with a disease model of mental illness rather than psychosocial goals. Addressing suicide, aggression, and psychiatric admissions is important to many personalized professionals learning goals. However, SDM on these topics is not

TABLE 6.4. Psychosocial Goals and Corresponding Interventions

Psychosocial goals	Manual title	Corresponding interventions
Support sustained recovery, reduce overdose risk, promote community integration	*Best Practices for Recovery Housing* (SAMHSA, 2023a)	Provide safe and supportive housing environments, offer peer support services, facilitate access to health care and employment resources
Promote successful reintegration, reduce recidivism, and address mental health and substance use needs	*Best Practices for Successful Re-Entry From Criminal Justice Settings for People Living With Mental Health Conditions and/or Substance Use Disorders* (SAMHSA, 2023b)	Develop individualized reentry plans, provide mental health and substance use treatment, and offer employment and housing assistance
Improve access to mental health and substance use services, address social determinants of health	*Expanding Access to and Use of Behavioral Health Services for People Experiencing Homelessness* (SAMHSA, 2023c)	Provide outreach and engagement services, offer integrated care in shelters and housing programs, address housing instability and basic needs
Enhance social support networks, promote recovery-oriented care	*TIP 64: Incorporating Peer Support Into Substance Use Disorder Treatment Services* (SAMHSA, 2023d)	Integrate peer support specialists into treatment teams, facilitate peer-led support groups, encourage mentorship and advocacy
Implement evidence-based policies to reduce alcohol misuse, promote public health	*Implementing Community-Level Policies to Prevent Alcohol Misuse* (SAMHSA, 2022)	Enact alcohol control policies (e.g., taxation, availability restrictions), educate community members on alcohol-related harms
Expand access to medication-assisted treatment for opioid use disorder, improve treatment outcomes	*Practical Tools for Prescribing and Promoting Buprenorphine in Primary Care Settings* (SAMHSA, 2021a)	Train primary care providers in buprenorphine prescribing, implement screening and brief intervention protocols
Prevent initiation of marijuana use among youths, reduce related harms	*Preventing Marijuana Use Among Youth* (SAMHSA, 2021b)	Implement school-based prevention programs, engage parents and communities in preventing marijuana use

Note. SAMHSA = Substance Abuse and Mental Health Services Administration. Adapted from *Evidence-Based Practices Resource Center*, by Substance Abuse and Mental Health Services Administration, n.d. (https://www.samhsa.gov/libraries/evidence-based-practices-resource-center). In the public domain.

grounded in *DSM-5-TR* (American Psychiatric Association, 2022) diagnoses. Understanding suicide, for example, does not necessarily begin with diagnostic differentiation of issues related to psychoses, mood, trauma, and multiple other co-occurring diagnoses. Rather, the SDM focal point begins with a careful behavioral and attitudinal analysis of the concern: What happens when you feel/are suicidal, or aggressive, or being hospitalized?

These manuals typically describe the problem (goal) and how it might be addressed. The manual on supported employment, for example, divides the enterprise into seven principles and practices to help people achieve their vocational and career goals. The tree begins with integrating supported employment efforts into the broader arena of personal mental health treatment. Real-world, and not sheltered, employment is the goal directed by personal preferences and rapid job searches. For instance, supported employment programs provide structured guidance on integrating vocational efforts into broader mental health treatment, emphasizing rapid job placement and ongoing support. Similarly, manuals addressing education-related goals focus on integrating mental health services into academic settings to help individuals succeed in their pursuits.

To avoid overwhelming individuals with too much information, summary trees provide a streamlined overview of key steps and actions. They also emphasize iterative processes in which individuals can revisit and refine their goals as they gain more clarity or encounter new challenges. For example, an individual pursuing a professional certificate might initially focus on enrollment requirements but later address barriers like mental health challenges or logistical concerns with the help of their provider.

Summaries must attend to information overload: Research has shown that too much information can overwhelm recipients and undermine their ability to make satisfactory decisions (Khaleel et al., 2020). PPLGs know best their information tolerance, which is likely to vary over time. Hence, summary trees provide a brief overview of information that, for instance, explains the process of returning to school (see Figure 6.4).

Other Resources

PPLGs might avail themselves of other resources to broaden their understanding of health conditions and psychosocial goals and interventions. The internet may be one good source, although caution is necessary here. Information from many sites may be influenced by a profit motive: to get people to purchase medications and devices or to buy a service. Two government entities have excellent search engines for health: the Centers for Disease Control and Prevention (see https://www.cdc.gov) and SAMHSA (see https://www.samhsa.gov). Especially notable on each site is a public information

FIGURE 6.4. Summary Trees for Organizing Summaries of Career Goals

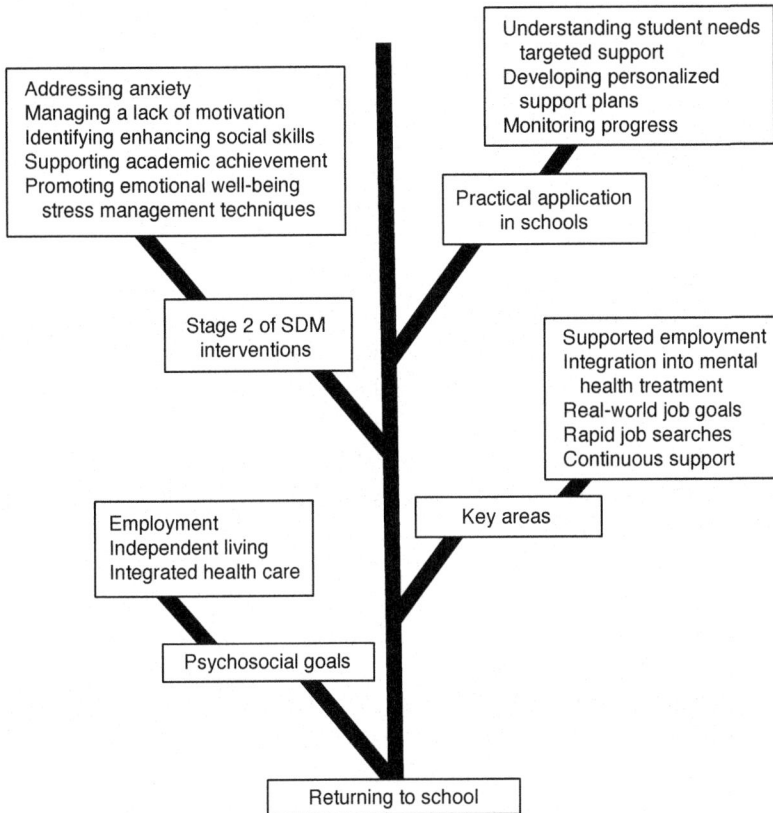

Addressing anxiety
Managing a lack of motivation
Identifying enhancing social skills
Supporting academic achievement
Promoting emotional well-being
  stress management techniques

Understanding student needs
  targeted support
Developing personalized
  support plans
Monitoring progress

Practical application
in schools

Stage 2 of SDM
interventions

Supported employment
Integration into mental
  health treatment
Real-world job goals
Rapid job searches
Continuous support

Employment
Independent living
Integrated health care

Key areas

Psychosocial goals

Returning to school

Note. SDM = shared decision making.

search engine PPLGs can use to type in questions about their health and wellness goals. WebMD (see https://www.webmd.com) is another resource with direct question search options; it is a private corporation sustained by ad sales, so there is some concern about whether content might be influenced by sponsors. Some nationally known clinics, including Mayo Clinic and Cleveland Clinic, also have publicly available resources. Professional associations (e.g., American Psychological Association, National Association of Social Workers, American Psychiatric Association), as well as advocacy groups (e.g., National Alliance on Mental Illness, Mental Health America, the Depression and Bipolar Support Alliance), also have websites that may be rich in information relevant to psychosocial goals.

We assume that more information helps the PPLG in the decision-making process with the aforementioned caveat about information overload. What, however, should PPLGs do if information from outside sources does not correspond with that from the P-SDM? This highlights an even broader role of P-SDMs: to help the PPLG sift through all information so the PPLG can develop a meaningful framework for them. In this role, P-SDMs need to suspend their own knowledge-based biases and help the person make sense of the total.

Step 4: Specify a Broad List of Actions to Achieve Goals

At this point, the PPLG and their provider have begun to gain a sense of personal goals with information about the nature of their condition or psychosocial goal as well as a menu of interventions and services that will help achieve these goals. Step 4 is turning those ideas into actions. Worksheet 3 summarizes those actions and composite tasks; it begins with another attempt to describe the focal goals of this SDM using information newly learned in Step 3 to fully unpack the issue. The PPLG makes an exhaustive list here of aspirations related to the central psychosocial goal. Returning to definitions based on information provided by the P-SDM provides another chance for the PPLG to step back and gain perspective. As always, the PPLG is encouraged to avoid static views of their goals; goals are often understood better as they address it over time.

At this point, PPLGs should avoid censoring ideas. Broad lists provide a grand vista of opportunities. Eight cells for actions are provided in Worksheet 3, although the PPLGs may identify more than eight, which could be entered on an additional worksheet. Actions listed in each cell include bulleted lists that address "what exactly": What exactly might the PPLG do to realize the specific action? The PPLG and P-SDM might have a collaborative discussion about actions as they are listed.

Example

Figure 6.5 is Fong's summary of actions that will help him get a professional certification that enhances his employability. He has outlined four actions. First, he needs to identify the field in which he wishes to pursue certification. He has values in terms of a career; a brief discussion with a career counselor will help him to better make sense of these values and then learn jobs that will help him live them out. Parallel with this action is understanding existing educational programs that lead to certification or license. Each of these will translate into a course of study, including the number of credit hours and years. This information will also lead to listing prerequisites. For example, what prior level of education is needed: a high school or baccalaureate degree?

FIGURE 6.5. Fong's Actions to Achieve Goals

Worksheet 3 Specifying Actions (and Tasks) to Achieve Goals

What are the key descriptors of either the focal health condition or psychosocial goal?

Health Condition	Psychosocial Goals
Symptoms •	Aspirations • Get a professional certificate
Other Constructs •	

What are all possible actions you might do to resolve your health condition or achieve your psychosocial goal? List specific tasks after every action	
Action #1 • Identify field • Gain a sense of various fields • What is the career trajectory for the field (any jobs out there) • What are the prerequisites • What are the curriculum demands (specific certification required for career shift/advancement	Action #5 • • • •
Action #2 • Identify program • What local school go to • Specific schedule Support cost	Action #6 • • •
Action #3 • Deal with mental health challenges • Learn about reasonable accommodation • Consider peer education navigators • What services does the student support center provide	Action #7 • • •
Action #4 • Home Support • How can family at home help • Family-centered decision making	Action #8 • • •

Is some formal testing required (e.g., the GRE)? Once career and certificate are identified, where might Fong go to pursue it? Is the program local, or would he need to move his residence? How much would the program cost? Are there academic support programs he might avail to offset this cost?

In discussing this plan, Fong better understood that his mental health challenges might interfere with enrolling, participating, and completing. How might he get a better sense of what specific challenges interfere with education? What accommodations might the program provide to help him deal with these challenges? What interventions does the student support service provide to support him through the challenges? Fong learned from the P-SDM, Leticia, about student peer education coaches. Does the school he chose have this? How exactly might peer coaches work? Fong lives at home with his parents. He wonders if and how they might support his education goals.

Step 5: Weigh the Pros and Cons of Options

In this step, the person–provider learning group evaluates the actions identified in Step 4 by weighing their pros and cons. This process is critical for determining which actions to include in the first draft of the comprehensive action plan (CAP) in Step 6. Worksheet 4 facilitates this evaluation by helping the PPLG analyze each action individually. The PPLG completes one worksheet for each of the actions listed in Worksheet 3. The PPLG begins by summarizing each action and explaining how it aligns with their overall goal. They then list all the pros and cons associated with the action. Pros are defined as ways in which the action helps achieve the goal, including ease of implementation and the availability of resources, whereas cons represent potential barriers or risks that might hinder progress toward the goal.

Although this assessment provides a comprehensive view of each action, the decision to include an action in the CAP is not based on a simple tally of pros and cons. Instead, a values clarification process is introduced to help PPLGs identify which pros and cons matter most to them. Some items may carry greater significance because of their alignment with personal priorities or values, and these should be circled or highlighted on the worksheet. This addition ensures that decisions are guided by what is most meaningful to the individual rather than an objective count of benefits and drawbacks.

Once this prioritization is complete, the PPLG reflects on the worksheet as a whole to determine whether an action should be included in the CAP. This holistic assessment allows for a nuanced decision-making process that considers both practical factors and personal significance. Collaborative discussion between the PPLG and their P-SDM often enhances this process by clarifying priorities and addressing uncertainties.

Example

Fong, a student returning to college while managing mental health challenges, evaluated "working with a student education coach" as a potential action. He created a pros-and-cons-of-action list (see Figure 6.6) and identified several pros, including access to personalized support, assistance from his school's student support center, and emotional support from Leticia. Among these,

FIGURE 6.6. Fong's Pros and Cons of Actions

Worksheet 4 Weighing Pros and Cons of Actions

Write down the specific action that corresponds with one goal	
Action(s)	Specific Procedure(s)
Obtain a career certification	Identify program or college Deal with the mental health challenge

Pros	Cons
☐ The school support center provides services ☐ I can seek help from Leticia Porter' ✓ A student education coach will be there to help me ☐ There are educational accommodations that can help me out ☐	☐ Going to school will stress me out ☐ I will feel all alone at school ☐ I will feel weak using the coach

Add to Action Plan

✓ Yes   ☐ No

Fong placed a check mark next to working with a coach as especially important because it aligned with his value of feeling prepared and supported. However, Fong also noted cons, such as increased stress from returning to school, feelings of isolation among peers, and potential shame associated with using peer coaches because of perceived weakness. Despite these concerns, Fong decided to include this action in his CAP because its benefits outweighed its drawbacks when viewed through his personal values.

Step 6: Make a Comprehensive Action Plan

Now it's time to put decisions into action. Worksheet 5 organizes actions selected in Worksheet 4 into a cogent plan to obtain the focal goal. This step is guided by Worksheet 5, which structures the plan around four key components: (a) what, (b) when, (c) who, and (d) measure of change. The "what" specifies the actions required to achieve the goal, the "when" outlines the timeline or sequence of actions, the "who" identifies those responsible or involved, and the "measure of change" defines how progress will be assessed. By addressing these elements, the CAP ensures clarity, feasibility, and accountability.

Example

Fong's goal of obtaining a career certificate (see Figure 6.7) only focuses on one action for the example. During Step 3, on fact-finding through expert

FIGURE 6.7. Fong's Comprehensive Action Plan

Worksheet 5 Developing a Comprehensive Action Plan (CAP)

Goal: Obtain a career certificate

Action 1: Identify the specific career, corresponding certification, and educational prerequisites

What	When	Who	Measure of Change

• Use information from Leticia to identify career values.
• Take a career interest inventory.
• Identify a career cluster that represents those values.
• Tentative chose one career designation.
• Identify certifications for a career.
• Identify educational institutions for training.
	• Need to do this sequentially
	  ○ Identify values,
	  ○ then a career,
	  ○ then a certificate,
	  ○ then a training program
	• Have some sense of the academic calendar and start dates.
		• Leticia will assist in the career assessment
		She will also help to search databases about
		  ○ Careers
		  ○ Certifications
		  ○ educational programs.
			• A clear decision on career
			• Clear decision certificate
			• A clear decision on the educational program.

Action 2:			
What	When	Who	Measure of Change

Action 3:			
What	When	Who	Measure of Change

Trying out the Plan
Beginning on: __/__/____ Going until: __/__/____

information, Fong learned about various career values and interests that can be assessed using career interest inventories, consultations with career advisors, and self-reflection. These individual approaches vary in terms of clarity, relevance to personal goals, and alignment with skill sets. Hence, a step before making a career choice may involve exploring and understanding personal career values and interests, leading to a clearer decision-making process. In this case, the actual career choice becomes Action 1 in the CAP. Fong has identified a specific career cluster that aligns with his values and interests. The "what" of this action includes researching various certifications associated with the chosen career path. Additional actions may involve identifying educational institutions that offer training programs relevant to the chosen career and understanding their prerequisites and start dates. To plan accordingly, Fong may need to consider the academic calendar and start dates for these programs. Subsequent actions for this CAP might include enrolling in a training program, completing the required coursework, and obtaining the necessary certification. These actions are outlined in subsequent steps of the CAP.

In terms of "when," these actions need to roll out in a stepwise fashion. First, Fong identifies career values that morph into vocational interests. This leads to identifying relevant certificate programs and educational institutions at which the certificate might be obtained.

Worksheet 5 also includes "Who," listing people involved in carrying out the specific action. Leticia is highlighted as "who" in several places in the plan. In most cases, Fong will be at the forefront of these actions with assistance from individuals, such as Leticia, career advisors, and educators. Leticia, in particular, will play a significant role in assisting with career assessment, researching careers, certifications, and educational programs, and the provision of support throughout the process.

PPLGs identify "measures of change," represent tangible evidence of career choice, certificate selection, and identification of education setting, in Column 4 of Worksheet 5. How will PPLGs know whether specific actions have any benefit? These are distinguished into process measures (e.g., Were individual components of the plan completed as outlined?) and outcome measures (e.g., Did the action improve PPLGs' lives by helping them accomplish some aspect of their goal?). Process measures answer questions like "Did Fong and support persons do what they said they would do in the plan?" Hence, assessment is straightforward; for Fong's Action 1—to identify career values, choose a career, and select a certification—the question is, "Yes or no: Were these steps completed?" Perhaps a more important and related process question is, "Is Fong actively pursuing the chosen career path?"

To answer questions like these, Fong might prepare some kind of tracking system, perhaps a checklist in which Fong checks off each milestone achieved in the career exploration and certification process. These checklists are more thoroughly developed in Step 7 on evaluating action plans.

Processes are only beneficial if they enhance outcomes. Did doing the act really make things better for the PPLG in terms of the focal goal? Three strategies might be appropriate for a health goal: symptoms, thoughts/affect, and biomarkers, explained in detail next:

Symptoms
Did symptoms diminish? Asking questions like this may be helpful. Mental health providers often think of standardized tests and outcome measures— for example, complete the Beck Depression Inventory (Beck et al., 1961) to determine whether the PPLG is less depressed. However, this can also be done more directly and efficiently. Assessing idiosyncratic target symptoms is one way: Idiosyncratic symptoms rest on a 100-point continuous scale from 0 (*noticing no symptoms*) to 100 (*as bad as the symptoms can get*).

A target symptom becomes idiosyncratic when PPLGs define scale anchors based on their personal experiences with the targeted symptom. For instance, Figure 6.8 represents the idiosyncratic target symptoms for Fong on the Idiosyncratic Target Symptom Scale (ITSS), on which he tracks his motiva-tion related to returning to school and obtaining a certificate (see Figure 6.9, which is an example of the ITSS). Fong views zero on the scale as the total absence of motivation. Things become noticeable at 25 on the scale, "feeling slightly interested in educational pursuits." Things are a bit more promising at 50 when motivation starts to increase, leading to active consideration of returning to school. The cap on the scale is 100 when motivation is at its peak with Fong fully committed to pursuing educational goals. There are no unequivocal definitions of scale items: Nothing all people would agree is an incontrovertible characterization of the low or high end of a scale. Rather, it represents an individual's perspective and experience.

The PPLG also needs to decide whether the time of day for completing an ITSS is important. For example, mental health symptoms—like motivation— may vary within individuals by time of day. PPLGs may report that their motivation seems to fluctuate throughout the day. Hence, at the least, PPLGs want to make sure to collect data on idiosyncratic target symptoms at the same time of day. More ambitiously, PPLGs may want to collect data on idiosyncratic target symptoms multiple times of day to obtain some sort of average for 24 hours.

FIGURE 6.8. Fong's Idiosyncratic Target Symptom Scale

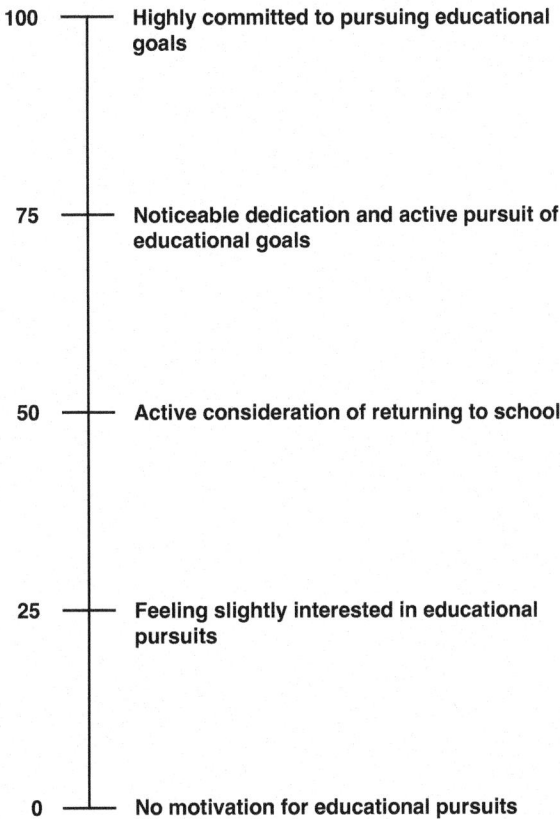

```
100 ──┬── Highly committed to pursuing educational
      │    goals
      │
      │
      │
 75 ──┼── Noticeable dedication and active pursuit of
      │    educational goals
      │
      │
      │
 50 ──┼── Active consideration of returning to school
      │
      │
      │
      │
 25 ──┼── Feeling slightly interested in educational
      │    pursuits
      │
      │
      │
  0 ──┴── No motivation for educational pursuits
```

Assessing Thoughts and Affect Related to the Goal

Successful outcomes are often associated with thoughts and emotions. Thoughts reflect such psychological variables as hope, self-efficacy, and self-determination:

- Hope: I am optimistic about my educational journey.
- Self-efficacy: I believe I have the capability to succeed academically.
- Self-determination: I am committed to achieving my educational goals.

Attitudes like this have an emotional feel to them that can be scored on a worksheet for idiosyncratic target symptoms: low versus high hope, self-efficacy, or self-determination. Instead of being target symptoms, PPLGs track target emotions. PPLGs anchor the five points of idiosyncratic target symptoms for these emotions (i.e., 0, 25, 50, 75, 100).

FIGURE 6.9. Example of Idiosyncratic Target Symptom Scale

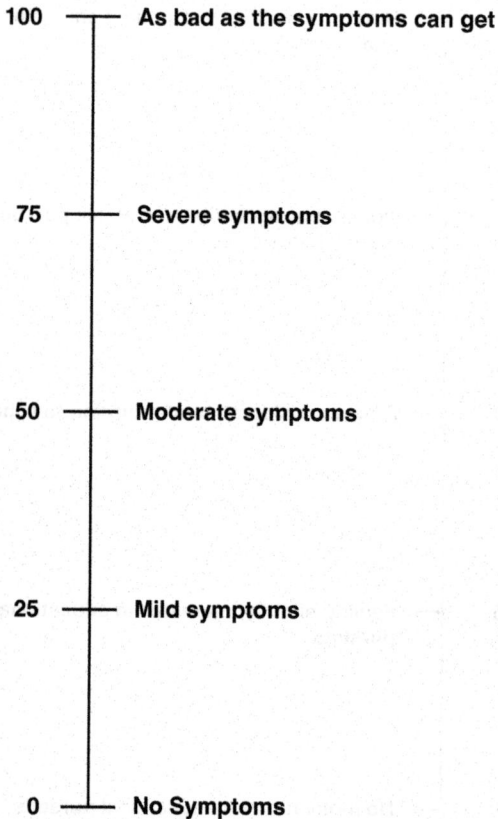

100 ——— As bad as the symptoms can get

75 ——— Severe symptoms

50 ——— Moderate symptoms

25 ——— Mild symptoms

0 ——— No Symptoms

Biomarkers

Findings from academic performance, for example, can represent the benefits of returning to school and obtaining a certificate. Fong may decide to regularly track his grades and academic progress. He can use these scores in a subsequent evaluation of the plan (see Step 7).

PPLGs and P-SDMs should step back after completing Worksheet 5 to view the plan as a whole. This may lead the PPLG to additional insights that add, omit, or revise individual actions. This should be a one-time revision; eventually, the PPLG needs to try it out. For this reason, the box at the bottom of Worksheet 5 proposes a window of time in which the plan will be attempted. The box includes a start date and an end date.

What happens if the P-SDM and PPLGs disagree on some aspect of the CAP? P-SDMs use their counseling skills to help the PPLG explore alternative decisions. P-SDMs suspend their expertise to help the person weigh the pros and cons of alternatives and select ones that best fit them. P-SDMs need to avoid any tone of professional authority that might undermine the person's complete self-determination of the CAP.

Step 7: Evaluate the Action Plan and Revise It When Necessary

PPLGs should attempt the CAP as outlined in Worksheet 5 with few changes to yield a fair test, that is, one that determines whether each action as planned leads to benefits. Hence, the test period should not be too long: Many have found about 2 weeks to be good. Yet, 2 weeks may not be enough time to notice change. For example, 2 weeks may be insufficient for career-related lifestyle changes to be noticeable; transitioning to a new study schedule and adapting to educational demands might not show significant results after only 2 weeks. Conversely, PPLGs may tire of the CAP if the test period is too long, especially if the CAP does not seem to be having any effect. That is why discussion about the Step 7 evaluation period is important. Despite requesting PPLGs to not veer from the CAP during the test period, PPLGs may avoid any part of the plan if they find it unexpectedly stress inducing.

PPLGs and P-SDMs should not expect the CAP written in Worksheet 5 to play out as planned or to lead to total success. This kind of a priori expectation avoids failure confirmations—"I knew this wouldn't work. Why did I even try?"—and helps PPLGs to be open minded during both framing the CAP (Step 6) as well as subsequent evaluation (Step 7): "What did I discover about myself and the psychosocial goal throughout the 2-week CAP?" Still, the purpose of the CAP is to yield insight about steps forward to the goal; it is a process over time. Worksheet 6 summarizes the evaluation step that helps the PPLG do this. It explicitly includes space for revisions to the plan that may emerge from the evaluation.

The PPLG transfers all the actions described in the CAP by number from Worksheet 5 to the corresponding cell of the evaluation Worksheet 6 along with their corresponding measures. The PPLG, perhaps with the help of the P-SDM, collects data related to these measures and then tries to determine whether the individual actions they took were beneficial and moved them toward their goal. Sometimes, the PPLG and P-SDM develop a separate summary sheet like the one in Worksheet 7 to track data as it occurs during the 2-week test period. The PPLG lists actions and corresponding measures in Column 1 of that worksheet. Then, they track behaviors or scores for each day of the 2-week trial. The goal, then, is to try to reduce scores in each box to a judgment about whether the specific goal was achieved. What does "achieved" mean here? It is not some sort of statistical process leading to a yes–no certainty of statistical significance ($p < .05$). Process judgments are a bit easier. The PPLG merely sums up whether the target behavior was done. Outcome judgments are a bit harder. Target symptoms might be used. The ITSS change is based on the 100-point Likert scale.

Unlike a basic statistics course, however, there is no t-test to determine whether the change in the ITSS is a true difference. An increase in ITSS scores suggests symptoms are getting worse, which is a bad sign that may require correction. But what kind of ITSS difference represents a benefit, a sign that movement toward the goal has been achieved? Does a 10-point drop on the ITSS representing depression suggest that symptoms are getting better? The P-SDM may discuss this with the PPLG at the beginning of a 2-week trial to help them get some sense of whether a score represents achievement.

This kind of discussion during the first few days often helps PPLGs get some sense of whether things are improving. Selecting "not sure" on the ITSS is an option. Measures that lead PPLGs to check frequent "not sures" suggest that future revisions of the CAP may require a new measure. PPLGs and P-SDMs sit down at the end of the 2 weeks and ask whether the CAP is working. If it is good as written, the PPLG is on their way toward achieving the focal goal and continues with the action plan. If substantial revisions are needed, a new CAP should be created, followed by another 2-week trial.

Example

Figure 6.10 shows the evaluation of the first action of Fong's CAP, namely, to identify a specific career direction, a certification program that will help him find a job in that area, and an existing education program. He listed six tasks in the CAP, including gathering information to identify possible career clusters, finding existing certifications related to those clusters, and identifying education programs that will help him earn the necessary certification. Measures were straightforward: evidence that the career, certification, and education program had been identified. Fong answered yes when Leticia asked if he had identified a career and certification but was unsure about a corresponding education program. Therefore, he proposed to revise the CAP by enrolling in and trying out a specific education program—at Olive-Harvey College—to see if it fit his goals.

GUIDELINES FOR FAMILY-CENTERED DECISION MAKING

As a Western approach to setting goals, SDM may require significant adaptation for collectivist cultures, such as those in many East and South Asian societies. In these cultures, individuals often prioritize the involvement of

FIGURE 6.10. Fong's Evaluation and Decision

Worksheet 6 Evaluate and Decide

When did the CAP begin? <u>October 28, 2023</u>

When is it to finish? <u>November 14, 2023</u>

Action (From Worksheet 5)	Measures	Achieved	Revise CAP
• Use information from Leticia to identify career values. • Take a career interest inventory. • Identify a career cluster that represents those values. • Tentative chose one career designation • Identify certifications for a career. • Identify educational institutions for training.	• A clear decision on career • Clear decision certificate • A clear decision on the educational program.	• Yes	Try out educational programs and evaluate at semester end

Action (From Worksheet 5)	Measures	Achieved	Revise CAP
		• Yes • No • Not Sure	• • •

Action (From Worksheet 5)	Measures	Achieved	Revise CAP
		• Yes • No • Not Sure	• • •

Action (From Worksheet 5)	Measures	Achieved	Revise CAP
		• Yes • No • Not Sure	• • •

Trying out the revised Plan
Beginning on: __/__/____   Going till: __/__/____

family members in decision-making processes. For example, the person participating in the life goals—the PPLG—may prefer that their family fully engage in and contribute to the decision-making process (Campos & Kim, 2017). Collectivist groups typically place high value on the opinions, beliefs, and actions of kin, family, or the broader community, which can sometimes result in decisions that reflect the collective preferences rather than solely those of the individual PPLG (Hofstede, 2011; Triandis, 2018).

In family-centered decision-making, family input may play a key role and could be integrated into the CAP. However, as with all aspects of SDM, it is ultimately up to the PPLG to decide who should or should not be included in the decision-making process. Although a practitioner of SDM (i.e., P-SDM) might assume that an individual PPLG prefers a family-centered approach, it is important to respect that the final decision about involving others rests with the PPLG.

Worksheet 8 summarizes components that inform choice about "family" in SDM. These considerations are typically made very early in SDM so PPLGs can work to include family members in the various steps. The worksheet begins with a yes–no question: Does the PPLG want family members to be included in SDM? This decision can be facilitated by P-SDMs discussing with the PPLG what family-centered decision-making entails. Key discussion points are as follows:

- Family-centered decision-making differs from how SDM is viewed in most of this book, which reflects a Western value. According to the Western perspective, PPLGs decide for themselves the goals and actions that will lead them to achieve their goals.

- Some PPLGs want family members to be included in the SDM process because of their cultural experiences. Family might be parents, partners, siblings, or adult children. This perspective is especially prominent in East Asian cultures, such as China or Japan.

- P-SDMs should not assume people from cultures other than East Asia do not value family-centeredness nor that all people from East Asia or similar cultures want to include families in their decision making. It is up to the PPLG to decide.

- To help the decision, PPLGs should consider how a family-centered approach would affect SDM. Briefly, one or more family members selected by the PPLG would fully attend and participate in selected steps of SDM. The PPLGs still have the option to change this strategy and exclude family—if they so decide.

PPLGs might find the act of completing Worksheet 8 informative regarding where they stand in terms of family centering. Eventually, though, it comes down to a yes–no decision: does the person want to include family in the process?

The family has a role in most PPLGs' decisions, whether family centered or not. PPLGs may identify specific family members to assist in specific steps of a CAP, but family members are somewhat removed from the decision-making process. Family-centered decision making suggests a different process. Selected family members are identified as active partners in the decisions at each step of SDM. Worksheet 8 asks PPLGs to list, by name, who in the family they would like included in SDM. Instead of "father," the PPLG should put down the name of their father to help the PPLG distinguish the ideal of one's father participating in SDM from the reality of their actual father. Family here might be anyone: parents or guardians, grandparents, siblings, adult children, extended family, and even friends or community leaders. There are presumptions of shared history and commitment. PPLGs select family members with whom they are regularly in contact and who have some sense of current needs on which the person is focused. Hence, PPLGs may wish to avoid a distant uncle they have not seen for years or a relatively new friend who does not have a sense of the person's life journey.

Family members who will engage in SDM need to commit to the process; namely, they join in all actions and tasks related to the steps as well as homework that follows from interactions. Conversely, PPLGs need to realize that family members they have identified on the worksheet may be unwilling to commit to the process. Hence, PPLGs need to inform family members about the seven steps of SDM so they know what they are agreeing to. PPLGs also need to consider the number of family members who wish to be included in family-centered decision making. Too many family members undermine the group process because too many opinions need to be balanced. Two to three might be a good maximum.

Worksheet 8 then asks PPLGs to select in which of the seven steps of the SDM process they want family members to participate in. Some PPLGs may decide against the default assumption of all seven, instead preferring family members to participate in a selected few. Choosing a subset of steps may be difficult because family members lack the perspective of what was decided in prior steps. The worksheet ends with some consideration of how decisions might be made. Discussion would seem to be basic to all possible processes. Something mechanical like a vote could then be chosen. Consensus, which is a more flexible approach to voting, is another option. The PPLG might choose unilateral decision making, either holding that power themselves or giving it to a single person, such as the father of the family. The decision here is not binding, but it helps PPLGs understand the varied ways in which their family might be included in the decision. PPLGs may reconsider this decision as SDM progresses.

Some characteristics of PPLGs might influence the family's role in SDM. For example, PPLGs with cognitive or social disabilities might find some individual steps difficult to accomplish. This may be especially apparent in working with older adults as they struggle with disabling conditions related to the dementia spectrum. In this case, roles are often reversed, and adult children might have a more active role in SDM. Still, participants need to be mindful of the empowerment and self-determination on which SDM rests. For example, the P-SDM as well as all family members need to make sure attitudes about cognition and aging do not lead to stigma that undermines the PPLG's central role in SDM.

The PPLG's primary spoken language might also factor in the family's role in SDM. People living in the United States whose first language is not English and who feel they are not conversant in the language may rely on family members to translate for them. In these situations, family members need to be clear about when they are serving as translators and when they are participating in family-centeredness.

The age of the PPLG is important, too, especially when the person is not a legal adult. The age of majority varies around the world from as young as 15 to 21 years old. Eighteen is the age across the United States. Parents or legal guardians have a legally mandated role in SDM. However, within these parameters, SDM varies by development stage. We encourage readers to review Chapter 4 in this book about how SDM appears in youths.

Example

After learning about family-centered decision making, Fong thought this was worth pursuing. He wanted to include his mother, Li, in the process. Fong currently lives at home with Li and felt she has been supportive and thoughtful about both his vocational exploration and about barriers to this journey caused by his mental health challenges. Figure 6.11 is Fong's completed family-centered decision-making worksheet on which he identified Li as the only participating family member and determined that he wanted her to be involved in all decision-making steps. He wanted the process to include decisions and consensus. The next step was for Fong to ask Li whether she wanted to participate in this process. Leticia might join Fong and Li in more fully explaining the expectations.

A CALL FOR FLEXIBLE SHARED DECISION MAKING

The SDM process as described in this chapter is long and comprehensive; it comprising many steps, actions, and tasks. Often, demands on the PPLG and the nature of the developing dyad might suggest a more selective approach in part because the PPLG does not have the time or motivation for such a large process. As PPLGs delve into the enterprise, they find some steps to be a distraction from the more pressing need to address their health

FIGURE 6.11. Fong's Family-Centered Decision Making

Worksheet 8 Considering Family Centered Decision Making

Do you want your family to be actively included in your shared decision-making?

(• Yes)   • No

Who in the family?	
Name: • Li Tsang •	Role in the family (eg-father, sister, brother, etc) • Mother •

What steps in SDM? (Check all that apply)

⊟-Step 1	⊟-Step 4	⊟-Step 6
⊟-Step 2	⊟-Step 5	⊟-Step 7
⊟-Step 3		

Decision-Making Process (What would you like family members to do?)	
• Discussion • _____ decides	• Consensus • I Decide

I can decide to change this form at any time

or psychosocial concerns. As a result, PPLGs and P-SDMs are encouraged to adapt the seven-step SDM plan to reflect a process that works best for the PPLG. This might include selecting worksheets that efficiently meet the focal goals. The dyad might also be selective within a step, only doing actions that seem relevant. Regardless of decisions, the PPLG and P-SDM should regularly circle back and ask whether their SDM process is meeting the focal goals.

CONCLUSION

This chapter has provided a comprehensive guide to implementing SDM in the context of mental health and psychosocial goals. It emphasized the importance of centering the process on the PPLG, ensuring that their values, aspirations, and preferences drive the decision-making process. The seven-step SDM framework, supported by practical tools, such as worksheets and summary trees, offers a structured yet flexible approach to identifying goals, exploring options, and creating actionable plans.

The chapter also highlighted the dynamic nature of goals, acknowledging that they evolve with new insights and changing priorities. The role of service providers (i.e., P-SDMs) was underscored as facilitators who guide the process by sharing expert knowledge, fostering collaboration, and respecting the PPLG's autonomy. Additionally, the inclusion of other stakeholders, such as family members or community leaders, was presented as an option that can enrich the process when aligned with the PPLG's preferences.

Recognizing cultural diversity and individual differences, the chapter advocated for adaptability in SDM practices, including family-centered approaches where appropriate. It also addressed potential barriers, such as information overload and logistical challenges, offering strategies to navigate these effectively.

Ultimately, this chapter serves as a practical road map for integrating SDM into mental health services, empowering individuals to take an active role in shaping their futures while fostering meaningful partnerships with providers and stakeholders. By grounding SDM in person-centered care and self-determination, it reinforces the overarching goal of supporting individuals in achieving both their immediate and long-term life aspirations.

REFERENCES

Agency for Healthcare Research and Quality. (2017, December). *The CAHPS ambulatory care improvement guide: Practical strategies for improving patient experience.* https://www.ahrq.gov/sites/default/files/wysiwyg/cahps/quality-improvement/improvement-guide/cahps-ambulatory-care-guide-full.pdf

American Psychiatric Association. (2022). *Diagnostic and statistical manual of mental disorders* (5th ed., text rev.). https://doi.org/10.1176/appi.books.9780890425787

Beck, A. T., Ward, C. H., Mendelson, M., Mock, J. E., & Erbaugh, J. K. (1961). An inventory for measuring depression. *Archives of General Psychiatry, 4*(6), 561–571. https://doi.org/10.1001/archpsyc.1961.01710120031004

Campos, B., & Kim, H. S. (2017). Incorporating the cultural diversity of family and close relationships into the study of health. *American Psychologist, 72*(6), 543–554. https://doi.org/10.1037/amp0000122

Dr. Robert Bree Collaborative. (2019, November 20). *Shared decision making* [Report]. Foundation for Health Care Quality. https://www.qualityhealth.org/bree/wp-content/uploads/sites/8/2019/11/Recommendations-Shared-Decision-Making-FINAL-2019.pdf

El-Harakeh, A., Morsi, R. Z., Fadlallah, R., Bou-Karroum, L., Lotfi, T., & Akl, E. A. (2019). Prioritization approaches in the development of health practice guidelines: A systematic review. *BMC Health Services Research, 19*(1), Article 692. https://doi.org/10.1186/s12913-019-4567-2

Elwyn, G., & Durand, M.-A. (2018, February 20). *Mastering shared decision making: The when, why, and how.* EBSCO. https://www.ebsco.com/blogs/health-notes/mastering-shared-decision-making-when-why-and-how

General Medical Council. (2020). *Decision making and consent* (Publication No. GMC/DMC/1224). https://www.gmc-uk.org/-/media/documents/gmc-guidance-for-doctors---decision-making-and-consent-english_pdf-84191055.pdf

Hofstede, G. (2011). Dimensionalizing cultures: The Hofstede model in context. *Online Readings in Psychology and Culture, 2*(1), Article 8. https://doi.org/10.9707/2307-0919.101

Khaleel, I., Wimmer, B. C., Peterson, G. M., Zaidi, S. T. R., Roehrer, E., Cummings, E., & Lee, K. (2020). Health information overload among health consumers: A scoping review. *Patient Education and Counseling, 103*(1), 15–32. https://doi.org/10.1016/j.pec.2019.08.008

National Institute for Health and Care Excellence. (2021, June 17). *Shared decision making: NICE guideline* (Publication No. NG197). https://www.nice.org.uk/guidance/ng197/resources/shared-decision-making-pdf-66142087186885

National Quality Forum. (2017, October). *Shared decision making: A standard of care for all patients* (National Quality Partners™ Action Brief). https://www.qualityforum.org/Publications/2017/10/NQP_Shared_Decision_Making_Action_Brief.aspx

NHS England and NHS Improvement. (2019, January 31). *Shared decision making: Summary guide* (Publication No. SDM Mini Guide v4). NHS England. https://www.england.nhs.uk/wp-content/uploads/2019/01/shared-decision-making-summary-guide-v1.pdf

Opel, D. J. (2018). A 4-step framework for shared decision-making in pediatrics. *Pediatrics, 142*(Suppl. 3), S149–S156.

Scottish Government. (2019, March 29). *Shared decision making in realistic medicine: What works.* https://www.gov.scot/publications/works-support-promote-shared-decision-making-synthesis-recent-evidence/

Shared Decision Making Collaborative. (2015, September). *A consensus statement.* Thrombosis UK. https://thrombosisuk.org/wp-content/uploads/2024/06/shared-decision-making-collaborative-consensus-statement.pdf

Substance Abuse and Mental Health Services Administration. (n.d.). *Evidence-based practices resource center.* https://www.samhsa.gov/libraries/evidence-based-practices-resource-center

Substance Abuse and Mental Health Services Administration. (2011). *Supporting choice: Helping others make important decisions. A step-by-step approach* (HHS Publication No. SMA-10-1124). U.S. Department of Health and Human Services.

Substance Abuse and Mental Health Services Administration. (2016). *Decisions in recovery: Treatment for opioid use disorders* (HHS Publication No. SMA-16-4993). U.S. Department of Health and Human Services. https://library.samhsa.gov/sites/default/files/sma16-4993.pdf

Substance Abuse and Mental Health Services Administration. (2021a). *Practical tools for prescribing and promoting buprenorphine in primary care settings* (Publication No. PEP21-06-01-002). https://library.samhsa.gov/sites/default/files/pep21-06-01-002.pdf

Substance Abuse and Mental Health Services Administration. (2021b). *Preventing marijuana use among youth* (Publication No. PEP21-06-01-001). https://library.samhsa.gov/sites/default/files/pep21-06-01-001.pdf

Substance Abuse and Mental Health Services Administration. (2022). *Implementing community-level policies to prevent alcohol misuse* (Publication No. PEP22-06-01-006). https://library.samhsa.gov/sites/default/files/pep22-06-01-006.pdf

Substance Abuse and Mental Health Services Administration. (2023a). *Best practices for recovery housing* (Publication No. PEP23-10-00-002). https://library.samhsa.gov/sites/default/files/pep23-10-00-002.pdf

Substance Abuse and Mental Health Services Administration. (2023b). *Best practices for successful reentry from criminal justice settings for people living with mental health conditions and/or substance use disorders* (Publication No. PEP23-06-06-001).

Substance Abuse and Mental Health Services Administration. (2023c). *Expanding access to and use of behavioral health services for people experiencing homelessness* (Publication No. PEP22-06-02-003). https://library.samhsa.gov/sites/default/files/pep22-06-02-003.pdf

Substance Abuse and Mental Health Services Administration. (2023d). *TIP 64: Incorporating peer support into substance use disorder treatment services* (Publication No. PEP23-02-001). https://library.samhsa.gov/sites/default/files/pep23-02-01-001.pdf

Triandis, H. C. (2018). *Individualism & collectivism*. Routledge.

U.S. Preventive Services Task Force. (2022). Collaboration and shared decision-making between patients and clinicians in preventive health care decisions and US Preventive Services Task Force recommendations. *JAMA, 327*(12), 1171–1176. https://doi.org/10.1001/jama.2022.3267

7

THE ROLE OF PARTICIPATORY RESEARCH IN REALIZING SHARED DECISION MAKING

LINDSAY SHEEHAN, RACHEL PARSON, AND CLARISSA VELÁZQUEZ

As previous chapters have demonstrated, shared decision making (SDM) provides an avenue for people with serious mental illness (SMI) to be involved in decisions regarding their life goals and the services that are available to them. In the spirit of SDM, interventions that promote SDM should be developed and implemented in collaboration with people who have lived experience with SMI. Furthermore, interventions should be applied, adapted, and evaluated in the context of local communities and specific populations (e.g., youths). The current chapter provides practical guidance for scholars and health professionals who wish to partner with the lived experience community in the design and development of SDM interventions by using a participatory research (PR) approach.

PR reflects a self-determined approach to research to actively include the perspectives and agendas of people with lived experience of recovery so that research findings reflect priorities of their lived community. This requires a paradigm shift in which people with lived experience are not subjects of research but, rather, partners in research. This chapter reviews how-to approaches to PR: ways in which PR teams can join together to better understand and implement SDM and self-determination. PR also has a significant

https://doi.org/10.1037/0000478-007
Shared Decision Making and Serious Mental Illness, P. W. Corrigan (Editor)

role in addressing social determinants of mental health when *community* is defined not only in terms of people with lived experience of recovery, but also as a socially constructed group that shares diversity (e.g., ethnicity, gender identity, sexual orientation) and marginalization (e.g., poverty, criminal justice involvement, immigration challenges).

TRADITIONAL VERSUS PARTICIPATORY RESEARCH PARADIGM

High-quality research is vital to the development, evaluation, and implementation of mental health services, treatments, and practices including SDM. Historically, health services research and medical research have been driven by the interests and priorities of academics and scientists rather than being centered around the needs and preferences of people who experience psychiatric conditions. In the traditional research paradigm, a scientist starts with a topic of their choice; identifies a research question (e.g., What personality traits are associated with the development of psychosis?); and selects research methodology largely based on their own experiences, expectations, and biases. These research questions may be well grounded in the context of the research literature and may lead to well-reasoned, logical hypotheses. However, these efforts may fail to have relevance to those who are currently experiencing mental health struggles. Furthermore, this paradigm fails to consider the perspectives of people with lived experience of SMI or capitalizes on their expertise in generating solutions and making changes in the mental health system. Just as the medical model of health care recognizes the physician as an expert who knows what treatment is best for the patient and views illness as a characteristic of the patient, the traditional research paradigm assumes that the scientist knows what is best for the community and that the scientist alone possesses the answers that will allow people with SMI to have meaningful lives.

Despite stigma, marginalization, and symptoms, people with SMI have organized a consumer movement that challenges the medical model of illness and emphasizes self-defined recovery and reforms within the health care system (Myrick & del Vecchio, 2016). This has included a surge in former or current service users who have taken on professional roles as mental health peer providers; developed evidence-based, peer-operated services; and taken on greater roles in research and advocacy (Mental Health America, n.d.). In parallel to the growth in peer providers, we have seen a growing emphasis on SDM in health care. SDM involves collaborative communication between a service user and their provider to jointly develop a plan centered around the service user's preferences and goals. In this chapter, we discuss how researchers and individuals with lived experience of SMI can use SDM in their research collaborations and how they can use PR to enhance health through SDM.

PARTICIPATORY RESEARCH DEFINED

Vaughn and Jacquez (2020) defined PR as an "umbrella term for research designs, methods, and frameworks that use systematic inquiry in direct collaboration with those affected by the issue being studied for the purpose of action or change" (p. 1). Per this definition, what differentiates PR from traditional research is collaboration with non–researcher community members and emphasis on change or action. Collaborations with those affected by the research topic—in this case, people with SMI—often take the form of community-based research teams that include individuals with lived experience of SMI. Ongoing collaboration with a lived experienced team allows opportunities for enhancing shared decisions throughout the research process itself and in the SDM intervention itself. For example, a researcher who has expertise in obsessive-compulsive disorder (OCD) might recruit a team of people who are living with OCD. This team would meet with the researcher regularly to collaborate on the systematic development and evaluation of an SDM intervention. The team's work might include conceptualizing the components of the intervention, conducting focus groups or interviews to guide development of the intervention, conducting pilots of the intervention, and selecting outcome measures for the intervention pilot. PR, as defined by Vaughn and Jacquez (2020), also emphasizes action or change. PR prioritizes research with a potential to have direct effects on individuals and communities. This is research that can be implemented or disseminated to improve lives or elicit changes. For example, an SDM intervention that includes the input of people with OCD may have more practical relevance to those living with OCD than those without. The individuals on the research team may then undertake implementation and dissemination efforts.

PR has been undertaken in a variety of disciplines, and there is a wide variation in the amount of direct collaboration (often called "engagement") with the community (see Vaughn & Jacquez, 2020, for a comprehensive list of approaches). Common frameworks and approaches to PR include participatory action research, community-engaged research (CEnR), patient-centered outcomes research, and community-based participatory research (CBPR).

These approaches all seek to involve marginalized groups from the community in research to effect social change.

Although we discuss levels of engagement more comprehensively later in the chapter, some types of research collaborations that may seemingly involve communities (e.g., community-academic partnerships) do not meet the definition of PR because they promote partnerships with community organizations (e.g., community mental health center leadership staff) but do not directly partner with lived experience individuals. Another related endeavor, *cocreation*, involves collaborations between professionals and the community to design materials, processes, or interventions. It may share many characteristics of PR, but it does not fall directly under the umbrella of research if the project does not include a systematic inquiry. Similarly, community-engaged program evaluations may use a similar process as PR but do not meet the definition of research.

BENEFICIAL OUTCOMES OF PARTICIPATORY RESEARCH

The research literature highlights a number of benefits to the implementation of PR, including benefits to the researcher, the lived experience of individuals involved in the research, and the broader community. We discuss these potential benefits in depth next.

Benefits to the Researcher

Frequent interaction with the community of people with SMI, as occurs in PR, helps academic researchers listen to and appreciate the lived experience perspectives. Greater awareness of the community, its resources, and the limitations of traditional research and service paradigms helps the researcher move into new research areas and develop partnerships for future research collaborations (Duran et al., 2019). The PR process will, ideally, over time, reduce the power differential that might exist between a provider and patient or researcher and community member. In this way, the researcher will learn how to share power, how to collaborate and communicate effectively, how to conduct research in more relevant ways, and how to initiate action based on research findings.

Historical and current unethical research practices have been perpetrated on both people of color and those with SMI, leading some in these communities to distrust researchers, the research process, and research findings. In psychiatric drug trials, people with SMI are paid to participate in research that results in immense profits to drug companies but that have significant side effects or disruption to their lives. For people of color, the Tuskegee study, in which effective treatment was withheld from Black men with syphilis (Brandt, 1978), remains a well-known barrier to participation of African Americans in research (Nooruddin et al., 2020). PR is one step toward building trust and relationships between science and the community, which can result in more sustained partnerships and synergize into multiple endeavors (Duran et al., 2019; Jagosh et al., 2015).

Benefits to Lived Experience Community Collaborators

When people with SMI experience stigma and disenfranchisement, that experience can result in feelings of resignation and the accompanying "why try" effect (Corrigan et al., 2009; Corrigan & Rao, 2012). In the why try effect, individuals with SMI may think, "Why even try to be involved in my community? Nobody cares about me anyway." PR provides an avenue for people with SMI to become catalyzed by their disenfranchisement and have power in transforming the system (Myrick & del Vecchio, 2016). Although some individuals who are former or current mental health service users (i.e., peers) have experienced empowerment through becoming professional peer health care providers or by participating in systems-level advocacy for mental health, PR provides another pathway for people with lived experience to make broader changes within the system. Involvement in PR can lead those with lived experience to enhance their social interaction, engage in meaningful activity, build work skills, and receive recognition within the community (Sheehan et al., 2021).

Benefits to the Community

PR challenges the assumptions of the traditional research paradigm by recognizing both collaboration with the community of affected individuals and social action as ethical imperatives (Case et al., 2014). This research is especially important when working with marginalized populations who experience the negative effects of *social determinants of health* (SDOH), which refers to nonmedical factors that affect health, such as education, income, and neighborhood environment (Compton & Shim, 2015). SDOH, which often stem from historical inequities in money, resources, and power, are seldom addressed by traditional health care and research systems. However, SDOH are increasingly recognized as having a vast influence on health disparities, which can be illuminated and addressed through PR. For example, a PR project was initiated in Seattle to address local inequities in asthma (Krieger et al., 2002). The PR team found that the physical deterioration of people's homes was the underlying cause for development of asthma. This revelation led to the community banding together to help restore some of the housing.

The marginalization of people with SMI has been long-standing, including physical segregation in residential settings, social exclusion, and the undermining of self-determination (Fakhoury & Priebe, 2007). Paternalistic attitudes and behaviors have often prevented people with SMI from participating fully in making decisions about their health care and their lives. Furthermore, stigma and marginalization have reduced their power in advocating for public health and research agendas that meet their needs (Bhui et al., 2006; Kidd & Davidson, 2007; Pelletier et al., 2009). From an ethical standpoint, PR practices in which individuals with SMI guide the work of academic research function as an anti-oppressive force to support social justice and address systemic health inequities.

Similarly, *intersectionality* refers to how individuals with multiple marginalized identities (e.g., an immigrant with SMI) are affected by oppression and develop solutions to address resulting disparities (Crenshaw, 1991). A recognition of intersectionality in PR helps ensure that projects aimed to help minoritized communities are being inclusive and that realistic solutions are implemented. PR projects that focus on intersectional populations (e.g., Puerto Rican women with posttraumatic stress disorder) should have team members from the community who reflect this same intersectional experience. For a PR project targeting youths with SMI, project leaders should have experience managing a group of youths; in addition, they need to decide how or if parents will be involved and how best to engage youths of the target age. Conversely, if a PR project is targeting older adults in an assisted living community, project leads might include health care providers on the team and make accommodations for physical and mental disabilities of team members.

Academic researchers are often siloed from their communities in a so-called ivory tower, conducting research in a way that lacks relevance to the community. PR improves the relevance of research when the individuals affected by SMI are involved in research, especially in the initial stages of selecting research topics and questions. This is more likely to result in research that is relevant to directly improving the lives of people with SMI. The relevance of results can help with translating these results into something useful for the community itself (Agénor, 2020).

Academic researchers often work within systems in which the needs of the university, health care system, or career of the researcher are often prioritized over the needs of the community. Academics and scientists have incentives to conduct research that leads to publication so they may achieve tenure and gain the esteem of their colleagues. University and health care systems have motives to bring in research grant funding and prestigious researchers but with limited consideration about how the community is affected. There is an overall lack of transparency in how research money is awarded, budgeted, and spent. Similarly, there is limited transparency in how research is conducted and how research participants are viewed by researchers. PR increases the transparency about research practices, opening more opportunities for research funds to benefit communities. For example, lived experience members of a PR team have opportunities to be paid for their work on the project and take on some tasks that would typically be done by a research assistant (e.g., recruiting, screening and interviewing participants). PR enhances the accountability of the researcher to finish projects, conduct research in an ethical way, and build awareness about how research can affect the community.

RESEARCH ON PARTICIPATORY RESEARCH

PR research has been increasingly supported by funders (Key et al., 2019). Since 2014, the U.S.-based Patient-Centered Outcomes Research Institute (PCORI) explicitly requires the health research that they fund to include collaborations with patients and stakeholders and has consistent funding opportunities for work that focuses on developing best practices for collaboration or engaging with patients. PCORI (2014) has an engagement rubric that guides academic researchers in partnering in the community in addition to a database of engagement tools funded through PCORI grants. The Institute of Medicine includes PR as a competency for all health professional students (Committee on Assuring the Health of the Public in the 21st Century, 2003), and the National Institutes of Health has developed extramural funding for PR projects (Tapp et al., 2013). Although efforts to measure engagement have proliferated in recent years, there is a need for study of why engagement in PR may lead to enhanced health outcomes and which methods of engagement are associated with the best outcomes for different stakeholder groups.

In an examination of 21 PR projects specific to mental health (funded by the National Institute of Mental Health), researchers and their community partners participated in surveys and interviews about their experiences (Khodyakov et al., 2011). This research found that levels of community engagement were associated with both perceived professional development and perceived community effects. Cross-sectional survey data from 200-plus federally funded investigators and 200-plus investigator-nominated community partners have been instrumental in developing validated measures for evaluating PR and connecting context and process variables to outcomes (Boursaw et al., 2021; Duran et al., 2019). As hypothesized, context and process-level variables explain variance in outcomes (Duran et al., 2019). For example, more reported power sharing within the team was associated with perceived improvements in community health. Similarly, the partnership capacity of the team was associated with more positive outcomes, whereas the mutuality of partners was connected with sustainability and community transformation. The findings highlight the importance of translation to practice—with the nature of PR (continuous collaboration and feedback) ensuring that research is connected to community needs and applications. Another analysis of these data ($n = 450$) found that partnership respect, influence in decision making, and stewardship predicted outcomes (Rodríguez Espinosa et al., 2020).

CONTINUUM OF ENGAGEMENT AND PARTICIPATION

Even within research that involves and engages communities, the level of direct community involvement varies by research project; thus, it is useful to describe participation or engagement as occurring on a continuum (Key et al., 2019). Inherent in the continuum model is the assumption that some community engagement is better than none. Figure 7.1 outlines six points along the continuum of community engagement from least to most involved according to the model by Key et al. (2019). Next, we describe and give examples of each of these: (a) community informed, (b) community consultation, (c) community participation, (d) community initiated, (e) CBPR, and (f) community driven.

Community Informed

At the community-informed level, the researcher incorporates information from the community into the research design. The community is not directly partnering, collaborating, or interacting with the researcher and may not even be aware that the community experience is being used to inform the research. An example of the community-informed level would be a researcher who

FIGURE 7.1. Continuum of Community Participation

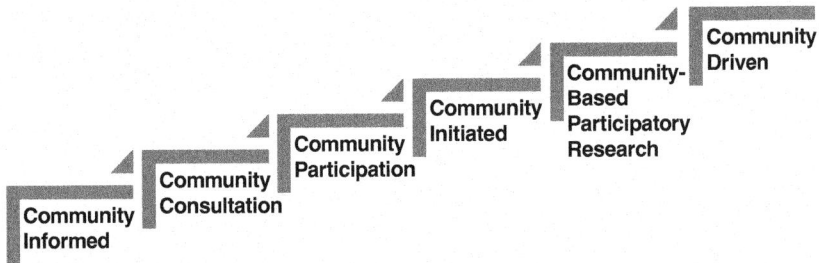

Note. Data from Key et al. (2019).

attends a community event and is inspired by a meeting, a speaker, or an informal conversation to pursue a particular research project. As such, this clearly does not meet the definition of PR.

Community Consultation

In community consultation, the researcher actively seeks feedback from the community to guide the research. Interaction between the researcher and community at this level is usually minimal and occurs at only one or two points during the research project. An example would be a researcher who presents their proposed project at a community organization and asks the community to share concerns or suggestions about the methodology, recruitment strategy, or effect on the community. This level also fails to meet the definition of PR because there is not a collaboration between the researcher and community.

Community Participation

At the level of community participation, members of the community have an active and defined role in the research project but are not involved in all aspects of the research project. In community participation, a researcher may recruit a community advisory board to provide ongoing (e.g., quarterly) feedback on the project or to help with a discrete task, such as data collection. This may meet the definition of PR provided that there is some level of collaboration and that collaboration is directly with community members who have lived experience of SMI or are in some way directly affected by the topic of study. However, participation at this level is often minimal and cursory, and the focus typically is not on research-based action.

Community Initiated

Community-initiated research occurs when a community member or community group approaches a researcher with a community priority that they would like to address through research. In this way, the community sets the research priority but may not be involved in the day-to-day decisions of the research study itself. This likely does not meet the definition of PR because there is not an ongoing collaboration.

Community-Based Participatory Research

In CBPR, there is shared ownership and team decision making between the researcher and community that occurs across time in multiple aspects of the research process. This clearly falls within the realm of PR. We discuss this type of PR extensively in the later section on CBPR; there, we provide a case example that depicts CBPR.

Community Driven

Community-driven research, or community-led research, involves community members who take full leadership of the research process. A traditional academic researcher may be involved in discrete tasks (e.g., data analysis) or may not have any involvement. In this way, the community has full ownership of the project and makes all decisions. An example would be a peer-run organization that decides to initiate a research project on employment for people with SMI and asks an academic researcher to give feedback on their research design and data analysis plan.

COMMUNITY-BASED PARTICIPATORY RESEARCH

CBPR is a type of PR that involves more intensive collaborations to provide community members with greater agency and involvement (Payán et al., 2022). CBPR arose with the purpose of addressing disparities and empowering marginalized communities (Israel et al., 2018; Minkler & Wallerstein, 2008). In Exhibit 7.1, we provide a case example of a CBPR project in which Dr. Diaz, an academic researcher, partners with service users and service providers to conduct a study on incorporating SDM into employment services for people with SMI. This case is a singular example of what CBPR might include. Each research project will be unique and will require flexibility to adapt to needs of the community partners, academic partners, and

EXHIBIT 7.1. Case Example: Community-Based Participatory Research

Dr. Diaz, an academic researcher, is invited to attend a recovery event at a local mental health center. While socializing with others at the event, one of the service users mentions their difficulties receiving employment supports that match their needs and preferences. Dr. Diaz has previously created and tested a tool to help doctors and patients engage in shared decision making (SDM) about psychiatric medications. She wonders if a similar tool could be used to help employment services staff at the mental health center incorporate SDM into employment-related services.

Dr. Diaz is aware of an upcoming grant opportunity that might fund this type of project. She reaches out to a staff member she knows at the mental health center to propose the idea and suggest a collaboration on a grant submission. Her initial contact is not in a leadership role at the organization but connects her with a program director, Chris, who has an interest in the project.

Dr. Diaz has a colleague who has done participatory research, and she seeks guidance from him. She decides on a community-based participatory research (CBPR) method. They advertise and hold a meeting at the mental health center for service users who may be interested. Dr. Diaz discusses her idea, asks for feedback, and invites the attendees to collaborate on the project. Sam, a service user from the agency's peer advisory board, is particularly interested in the project, and Dr. Diaz invites them to have a leadership role on the project.

Dr. Diaz writes and submits the grant. Ten months later, she lets the collaborators know that the grant is funded, and they begin planning meetings. Dr. Diaz, Sam, and Chris meet to map major goals for the project and recruit the rest of the team. They reach out to service users who were previously involved in the brainstorming session and invite them to participate as team members. They also post a flier in the mental health center to see if other service users are interested in joining the team. Once they have received a commitment from six service users, they schedule weekly meetings for which service users are paid for their time. They start with discussing roles, expectations, and ground rules for the team. Next, they complete training on CBPR and research ethics and discuss the research protocol. Dr. Diaz presents a literature review on the topic and discusses evidence-based components of previous SDM interventions. The service users on the team discuss their lived experiences with pursuing employment and how SDM might be incorporated through employment services.

The team decides to conduct research interviews with employment services providers and users around use and preferences for incorporating SDM into employment planning. Then, based on the interviews, they plan to conduct a larger survey on SDM in employment. They will use the results of their research to develop an SDM tool.

The service users help with preparing the recruitment materials and informed consent for research participants. Service users are included on the institutional review board submission. A few service users are trained to conduct interviews. The team meets weekly for the first 2 months of the project and then monthly thereafter during data collection. Once data are collected, the team convenes to make sense of the data and how to incorporate data into the SDM tool. They begin meeting more frequently to develop the tool and to work on developing a paper and presentation about their research. Team members are invited to be authors on papers and presentations. The team decides to present their work at the annual mental health gala.

Note. Case examples in this book are hypothetical.

environmental context. To guide implementation of CBPR, scholars have identified core principles to consider when planning CBPR projects. These principles are outlined in Table 7.1 and are accompanied by examples from the case example. Importantly, these principles guide rather than proscribe how CBPR should unfold.

In the principles shown in Table 7.1, words such as collaboration, team, partnership, iterative, and bidirectional highlight the interactive nature of the CBPR endeavor and the importance of SDM within the CBPR process itself. Although CBPR can be initiated by either a researcher or community member, a core feature is that the research focuses on issues relevant to

TABLE 7.1. Core Principles of Community-Based Participatory Research and Examples From Case Example

Principle	Examples from case example (see Exhibit 7.1)
Equitable collaborations occur during entire research process	The team is involved from conceptualization to dissemination
The team identifies and defines a specific community of interest	*Community of interest* is defined as people with mental illness who are receiving employment services
The project addresses marginalization of identities, intersectionality, or social determinants of health	People with mental illness are stigmatized in employment and may not be empowered during the employment process; SDM addresses this marginalization
Teamwork builds on the strengths of the community and each member of the team	Service users and providers each understand SDM process from their unique perspective; research brings expertise in SDM research
Interaction among the team includes bidirectional learning and is iterative in nature	Service users have a chance to share their perspectives and teach the researcher about their community while also learning about research
The work of the team maintains a balance between research and action for the mutual benefit of the team	Research data are collected and used for creating a tool that can enhance SDM in real-world settings
The process empowers the community in decision making	Service users from the community are involved at decision points in the research
Research focuses on issues relevant to the local community	Research was initiated in response to a community-identified problem
CBPR develops partnerships, systems, and capacity for future efforts	The team relationship may lead to new projects over time; the team could apply for funding to test the tool or could work on implementing it with the health center

Note. CBPR = community-based participatory research; SDM = shared decision making. Data from Israel et al. (2018).

the community and there is both research and community action contained within project goals. CBPR is meant to focus on the strengths of the community, addressing inequities in the health system. It is important here to emphasize an overarching aspect of any PR: translation to practice. The importance of involving community members is to ensure that interventions or research practices are consistently relevant to the needs of the community, that those interventions or research practices remain connected to real-world applications, and that findings are implemented in practice. The seventh principle emphasizes the empowerment and community involvement in decisions on the project. Later, in the section "Shared Decision Making: An Object of Community-Based Participatory Research at Each Research Stage," we explore further how SDM can be implemented within the CBPR team itself.

The Inspiring Change Model of Community-Based Participatory Research

One conceptual model of CBPR, called inspiring change, was originally developed to guide research for an intersectional group, African Americans with SMI, and then adapted more broadly for multiple intersectional identities (Sheehan et al., 2016). In the inspiring change CBPR model, an academic researcher, a health care service provider, and an individual with lived experience of SMI form a leadership triumvirate that guides the initial stages of the project. Together, they recruit a larger team, much as described in our case example (see Exhibit 7.1) and shown in Figure 7.2.

The inspiring change framework maintains that individuals with lived experience of SMI should not only be members of a CBPR team but also take on leadership roles. Thus, our CBPR model includes a research team led jointly with a service user. The inspiring change curriculum guides teams in collaboratively planning research and engaging the team throughout the research process. This team model requires the three team leaders to dynamically interact and manage individuals in a group. The team starts by developing ground rules for the team, examining issues of power sharing, and learning about the principles of CBPR together. A workbook provides discussion questions, worksheets, and brainstorming activities that allow the team to learn about CBPR and develop their research plan in an interactive way. The team is guided through decision points in the process, such as selecting a research topic, research questions and methods, and dissemination of results.

The academic researcher brings the expertise to ensure that projects are scientifically rigorous and adhere to standards of research ethics. In this way,

FIGURE 7.2. Inspiring Change Model of Community-Based Participatory Research

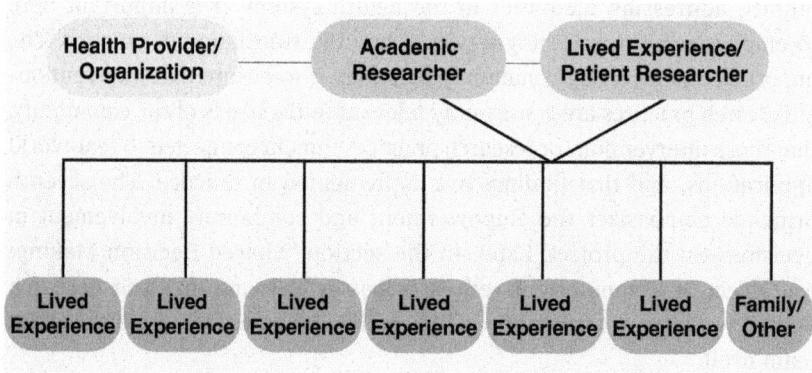

Note. Data from Sheehan et al. (2016).

the academic researcher serves as a bridge between the rest of the CBPR team and the scientific community. The health care provider brings insight from both the lived experience and health care perspectives to advise how research protocols might be received by health care administrators and how the results can be most widely disseminated in health care settings. Likewise, the lived experience patient research leader brings knowledge of how the research might be received by the community and how the team can best engage the other CBPR members throughout the research process. This lived experience leader serves as role model, advocate, cultural translator, and barometer for the engagement of community and participants. Together, the three project leaders develop a preliminary research plan and recruit a CBPR team of people with lived experience and other stakeholders to further develop and implement the research plan. The leadership team (i.e., academic researcher, health care provider, and patient researcher) are part of the larger CBPR team, which includes service users with lived experience.

The lived experience leader has a vital role in engagement. They help build trust within the team, help convey information in an understandable way, and ensure that the patient CBPR members are each able to contribute to the project in meaningful ways that highlight their strengths. These contributions are individualized, and the lived experience leader must learn to recognize individual strengths and match these to tasks that need to be accomplished. The lived experience leader emphasizes the importance of each contribution and must fully engage within the group setting. The inspiring change CBPR curriculum also includes a training curriculum for experienced leaders.

Shared Decision Making: An Object of Community-Based Participatory Research at Each Research Stage

SDM is merely a metaphor for what CBPR looks like in a research setting, and PR branches from CBPR. CBPR is a parallel process to PR, not an object of SDM. Like CBPR, PR is largely based around the idea of reducing power dynamics in the research team by encouraging collaboration between the investigators and community members. Additionally, like CBPR, PR increases community determination for itself in that the community team members and the investigative team work together to determine the needs and problems of the community. Both the community and research team collaborate to come to a solution to address the problems and needs in the community. However, trying to conceive all moving parts of PR and incorporating SDM can be overwhelming.

For the PR novice, it may be difficult to consider how and when in the research project decision making can be accomplished within the research team. Within each research stage are points when decisions must be made; at each point are myriad ways in which that decision could be made (Vaughn & Jacquez, 2020). For example, in deciding on a methodology, the researcher could decide themselves and present this idea to the team for feedback, present multiple research methodologies to the team for discussion, or ask team members to suggest research methodologies. One qualitative study of the PR process in people with SMI found that PR teams use various strategies for making research decisions on their projects (Sheehan et al., 2021). These included deferring to the person with expertise to make the decision, the leaders deciding with or without team input, the team discussing and coming to a consensus, or taking a formal vote. PR team members in that study also highlighted the need for conflict resolution as related to decision making.

Table 7.2 depicts opportunities for decision making with the team and the questions that might be asked during team research meetings at each stage in the research project (i.e., partnership development, study design, data collection, data analysis, dissemination, and implementation/action). In the partnership development stage, the team is developing shared goals

TABLE 7.2. Opportunities for Shared Decision Making at Each Research Stage

Partnership development	Study design	Data collection	Data analysis	Dissemination	Implementation and action
What are our shared goals and objectives?	What are our research questions and hypotheses?	How do we address emerging challenges with recruitment?	What preparation does the team need to understand the data?	How will results be disseminated to the research community (e.g., academic presentations, publications)?	How can the findings be implemented in the community?
Do we want to work together at this time?	Who will we collect data from?	Are adjustments needed to timeline or budget?	How will the data be presented and discussed within the team?	How will results be disseminated to the target community (e.g., community presentations)?	What actions might we take in response to the research findings?
Who else should we invite to be part of the project?	What research method will we use (i.e., qualitative, quantitative, mixed)?	What changes are needed to the protocol in response to preliminary data collection?	How are the findings relevant to the target community (from the perspective of the team)?	How will each member of the team be involved in dissemination efforts?	What are we able or willing to do now regarding implementation or action?
What is our timeframe for the project?	How will we recruit research participants?	Are our research participants properly supported and connected to resources?	How do we describe or discuss unexpected findings?	Who else (outside the team) might be involved in dissemination efforts?	Who and how will each team member be involved in implementation or action?

How will we make decisions on the project?	How will we ensure that our research is conducted in an ethical and culturally responsive way?	How do we retain participants in the study?	What further research questions are generated based on the current findings?	How will authorship for presentations or publications be shared?	What might be later steps for implementation or action?
What are our respective roles and responsibilities on the project?	How many participants will be included in the study?	How will the research team be involved in data analysis?	How does what we found fit within the context of other research?	Is additional funding needed? What are additional sources of funding to pursue?	
What are the most important outcomes for this project?	How will research team members be involved in data collection?	Do the preliminary data suggest needs for future data collection or community action?	Which findings will we focus on?		
How do we want this project to affect the community?	Will we compensate research participants? If yes, how?		What will the team or partnership look like moving forward (next steps for research)?		
How will members of the team be compensated?	What is the timeframe for data collection?				
How will we evaluate our partnership in ongoing way?	How will we address potential biases in research?				

for the project while making decisions about roles and responsibilities of team members. Partnership development usually begins with a core group and expands to include additional individuals. Decision making at this stage sets the tone for future decisions. Similarly, the study design phase includes many key decision points that persist throughout the project and set a precedent for engagement. The team may wish to select research methods that lived experience individuals can more easily understand, participate in, and interpret (Vaughn & Jacquez, 2020). Data collection and analysis are stages during which there may be fewer opportunities for SDM within the team, and the team may meet less frequently. Lived experience and community members may again have an increased role once the project moves into the dissemination and action phases.

GENERAL ENGAGEMENT STRATEGIES IN PARTICIPATORY RESEARCH

Researchers and health care providers benefit from preparation on how to engage with the PR team. To address power dynamics, those with more social power in the research group, like non–community research team members, may take particular care to reduce how much they talk in meetings to encourage all community members to participate and share their opinions. Researchers are encouraged to take off their "researcher hat" and providers to take off the "provider hat" and to view the individuals with lived experience as colleagues. The researcher should be mindful of using technical jargon and be prepared to explain concepts in multiple ways to ensure the team's understanding of research methods. All leaders can explicitly encourage critical feedback and provide team members with agenda materials in advance.

The meetings should be held at a consistent time and at a location that is convenient and comfortable for community members. Especially in the first several meetings, time can be reserved for some sharing of relationship-building activities, such as personal check-ins or icebreakers. Team leaders should be sure to provide prompt compensation and regular communication and to seek regular feedback from the team about the PR process. Vaughn and Jacquez (2020) provided an overview of existing engagement tools that can be useful at different stages during the research process. For example, during the dissemination stage, they highlighted a mapping system (Driedger et al., 2007) and ethnodrama tool (Taylor et al., 2017). PCORI (n.d.) also maintains a database of engagement tools created through their funding mechanisms.

USE OF A PARTICIPATORY RESEARCH APPROACH TO TEST AND IMPLEMENT SHARED DECISION MAKING

SDM involves an interaction between service user and provider to help the service user communicate their health goals, discover the options to address these goals, and collaboratively develop a treatment plan. Although SDM has been widely researched and promoted in the mental health field, it continues to lack full adoption in health care settings, and surprisingly little research on SDM has been done in a participatory way. Despite this, there is an increase in the interest in implementing SDM interventions in psychiatric settings. A successful implementation of SDM in a mental health setting occurred when a PR team assisted in developing SDM intervention for psychiatric medication use (Mahone et al., 2011).

Although SDM has been successfully implemented in psychiatric settings, there are still challenges to adopting SDM. Barriers to successfully implementing SDM may be more effectively addressed through PR because PR parallels the collaborative process of SDM. An important pillar of PR is engaging communities in the process of research, including procedures for successful communication and decision making with researchers while balancing the power dynamic between parties (Collins et al., 2018). In this way, PR brings relevant stakeholders (e.g., health providers, service users, managers) into an equitable collaboration that identifies and addresses the SDM barriers from multiple perspectives, ensuring that responsibility, ownership, and commitment to implementation are shared (Grande, Durand, et al., 2014).

CHALLENGES IN PARTICIPATORY RESEARCH

Although PR is a promising type of research, various challenges may arise during PR implementation. These include general challenges, such as scarcity of resources; challenges specific to the researcher, such as conflicts among the research team and the academic team; and challenges related to the health care provider or clinical team members, such as the demanding commitment of participation. Next, we discuss in detail how to recognize and address these challenges.

General Challenges

We organize general challenges of PR into several categories. They are power sharing; dual relationships; lived experience researcher protections;

resources, compensation, and institutional barriers; and preparation and training.

Power Sharing

People with lived experience often enter projects with clear disadvantages in terms of social power, education, and research experience, which may cause them to become frustrated or disengaged or to exist primarily as token participants. First, people with lived experience are transitioning from a role of service recipient with an inherent power imbalance relative to the researcher and health care provider. Researchers must openly acknowledge this power imbalance, and lived experience team members must navigate this power imbalance and transition into the role of partner rather than recipient. This requires the person to identify and develop their strengths going into the project and become confident in the important role that they will provide on the research team. This also requires team members with lived experience to communicate with the researcher to ensure their voices are reflected in the project. Experiences of racial discrimination and stressors related to working in unfamiliar or White-dominated environments could compromise the confidence and effectiveness of lived experience collaborators. Involving multiple individuals who share the marginalized identity and having at least one of those in a leadership position may reduce tokenism and power differentials (Sheehan et al., 2022). Lived experience team members, despite being in recovery, may still experience periodic psychiatric symptoms or require reasonable accommodations. This could require, for example, extra support from other leaders in planning or structuring of research tasks or debriefing after team sessions.

Second, people with SMI might be at a disadvantage in terms of formal education and experience with the basics of conducting research. People with SMI have important knowledge to bring to projects but can misunderstand or misinterpret jargon used by researchers. The researcher must create an environment in which lived experience team members are able to directly acknowledge any lack of understanding and seek clarification. If information conveyed by the researcher and provider is not expressed in words that a nonresearcher would understand, then the spirit of PR is not preserved, and the research risks losing a culturally competent approach.

Dual Relationships

Dual relationships occur when a PR team member has a relationship with another team member or research participant that occurs outside the work of the PR team. Although dual relationships may be more common in rural areas, in small cultural communities, or for projects embedded within community organizations, they are likely to happen during any PR project. The researcher may know individuals with lived experience through shared community affiliations or previous research projects (Souleymanov et al., 2016). A health care service provider may work for an organization from which a team member receives services. Individuals from the team may form relationships over time. A shared understanding of the nuances of dual relationships should be discussed at the outset of the group and monitored over time. Although a team member providing direct services to another team member is clearly problematic, other dual relationships may be appropriate provided that boundaries are appropriately managed.

Lived Experience Researcher Protections

Although lived experience individuals working on PR teams are not considered research participants and are not under the purview of the institutional review board (IRB), there are nevertheless protection concerns. When community members with lived experience are involved in data collection, a high level of training, support, and oversight is needed to protect individuals from traveling in unsafe neighborhoods, interacting with difficult participants, or responding to research participants in distress (True et al., 2017). Lived experience researchers may experience stress from interacting with research participants and risk having unfair burdens of data collection placed on them.

Resources, Compensation, and Institutional Barriers

Individuals with lived experience may struggle to understand and navigate academic and health care culture and norms and lack access to resources. Collaborators with lived experience who are not usually employees of the agency may lack resources, such as office space to store paperwork, access to electronic room scheduling, authorization to use computers or copy machines, or other privileges of employment. Other employees of the agency may fail to recognize or understand their role, which can erode the confidence of the lived experience leader. Organizations need guidance and training on how to incorporate PR needs into financial and research oversight structures (e.g., allowing community members to complete IRB training and be involved in data collection; Souleymanov et al., 2016). Because of limited experience working in academic research settings, lived experience team members can benefit from extra support in navigating effectively in professional work environments and advocating for organizational resources and support. Similarly, because of their nonemployee status, lived experience team members may be paid differently than the service provider and research leaders (e.g., gift cards versus paychecks). This difference in pay can potentially undervalue the patient leader's contribution to the project and allow the leader to view themselves more as a research participant than a research partner (Guta & Voronka, 2020).

Preparation and Training

Researchers who wish to initiate a PR project for the first time will benefit from preparation and training. Typically, researchers are not trained in how to develop partnerships in the community, manage the dynamics of a team, or engage in this level of ongoing collaboration. Although most universities and health systems have a designated office or staff who manage community relationships, these rarely provide support in terms of specific trainings for engaging in PR. However, these offices may provide support in suggesting partnership opportunities. Universities increasingly are offering courses in PR, although those offerings are still rare. The aforementioned inspiring change curriculum provides a hands-on primer for PR.

Each project faces different challenges, and having a mentor, especially within the same institutional setting, who can help with managing institutional barriers can be extremely valuable. Individuals with lived experience and other stakeholders who might want to be in leadership roles may need training in office skills, computer literacy, or group leadership before they take on these roles. In most cases, community members working on PR projects are not trained extensively in research methods. The researcher, who has expertise in research methods, can present an overview of the research methods as necessary to complete the specific project.

Challenges Specific to the Researcher

Because of the level of community involvement, a PR project is often of longer duration, especially during the planning and development stage. The researcher should allow sufficient time for this and will need to exercise patience with this process. Initial partnerships may not come to fruition, or interpersonal conflicts can derail the project. Thus, PR projects require a high level of interpersonal skill and understanding of group dynamics to ensure the continued engagement of all members of the team.

The researcher needs to be organized and proactive in addressing challenges. These efforts include developing agendas for each meeting and sending out meeting materials for review, ensuring that team members are paid in a timely way, and liaising with administration about IRB and payment issues that are specific to PR. To compensate the team, the researcher must plan in advance to include enough funding in the budget over the course of the project and find other sources of funding to maintain the partnerships over time. Researcher efforts in PR are not always recognized in the tenure and promotion process (rather, the focus is on grants and publications), so there are systemic disincentives to engage in PR.

Challenges Specific to the Health Provider or Clinician Team Member

The inclusion of a health care provider on PR projects that address health disparities can be extremely valuable to the project outcomes, especially regarding feasibility and implementation when there are barriers to participation for the health care providers. By the nature of their occupation, these providers are occupied with providing services and often have limited time to devote to research (Wallerstein & Duran, 2006). They may be primarily concerned with immediate community improvement and become frustrated with a lengthy research process. Research methodology, such as randomized clinical trials in which only some patients can access services or can access only time-limited services can be frustrating to clinicians (Wallerstein & Duran, 2006). The team leaders need to keep these limitations in mind when partnering with clinicians and attempt to work around these challenges.

EVALUATION OF PARTICIPATORY RESEARCH

Despite a growth in PR approaches supported by funders in recent years, collaborative research can be challenging to implement, especially in historically marginalized or medically underserved populations (Payán et al., 2022; Wallerstein et al., 2019). At the core of these challenges is engagement: the development of reciprocal partnerships between researchers and community members that are based in transparency, trust, honesty, and bidirectional learning (PCORI, 2014).

The Donabedian Framework

The Donabedian framework (Donabedian, 1988) was developed as a measure of quality of care in clinical health care settings but can be applied to the evaluation of PR. The framework includes three components: (a) structure/ context, (b) process, and (c) outcome.

Structure/Context

In CEnR, structure/context includes constructs such as readiness for research, amount of funding, institution type, research method, and population of study. It also includes confidence or motivation or attitudes, strengths and resources of the community, past experience, and level of training in PR (Boursaw et al., 2021; Luger et al., 2020).

Process

Process measures include those that capture the relationship among team members. These measures include trust, transparency, mutual respect, group dynamics, partnership, communication, power sharing or SDM, and role clarity.

Outcome

Outcome measures may include the capacity for future research. They also may include community translation of research findings, dissemination, empowerment of team members, and skills or knowledge acquired (Boursaw et al., 2021; Luger et al., 2020).

Engagement Scales and Measures

Some large-scale research has produced valid measures and testing of hypotheses around how context and process variables can predict outcomes (Boursaw et al., 2021; Duran et al., 2019). For evaluating individual PR projects, several measures with adequate reliability and validity have been provided by Boursaw et al. (2021). Other evaluation tools include the Group-Level Assessment (Vaughn & Lohmueller, 2014) for assessing context and the Community Engagement Measure (Goodman et al., 2017) for measuring process variables. The Critical Outcomes of Research Engagement (Dillon et al., 2017) and the Learning Outcomes of Community-Based Research (Lichtenstein et al., 2011) are among the available outcome assessments for PR. Some of these scales can be administered to the team during various points in the research process with results fed back to the team for continued improvement.

CONCLUSION

PR offers significant potential to advance research on SDM. This chapter introduced the concept of PR, exemplified through a case example that demonstrated the core principles of CBPR. We proposed methods for research teams to use PR to fill research gaps and provided guidelines for engaging stakeholders in PR. Additionally, we discussed common challenges in PR and suggested models for its implementation.

Clearly, implementing PR is a complex process that necessitates long-term development of robust community partnerships and structural changes (Vaughn & Jacquez, 2020). Those who wish to engage in PR should thoroughly examine their motivations, adhere to the foundational principles of PR, ensure their project remains true to these principles, and develop strategies to assess engagement throughout the process.

REFERENCES

Agénor, M. (2020). Future directions for incorporating intersectionality into quantitative population health research. *American Journal of Public Health, 110*(6), 803–806. https://doi.org/10.2105/AJPH.2020.305610

Bhui, K., Shanahan, L., & Harding, G. (2006). Homelessness and mental illness: A literature review and a qualitative study of perceptions of the adequacy of care. *The International Journal of Social Psychiatry, 52*(2), 152–165. https://doi.org/10.1177/0020764006062096

Boursaw, B., Oetzel, J. G., Dickson, E., Thein, T. S., Sanchez-Youngman, S., Peña, J., Parker, M., Magarati, M., Littledeer, L., Duran, B., & Wallerstein, N. (2021). Scales of practices and outcomes for community-engaged research. *American Journal of Community Psychology, 67*(3–4), 256–270. https://doi.org/10.1002/ajcp.12503

Brandt, A. M. (1978). Racism and research: The case of the Tuskegee Syphilis Study. *The Hastings Center Report, 8*(6), 21–29. https://doi.org/10.2307/3561468

Case, A. D., Byrd, R., Claggett, E., DeVeaux, S., Perkins, R., Huang, C., Sernyak, M. J., Steiner, J. L., Cole, R., LaPaglia, D. M., Bailey, M., Buchanan, C., Johnson, A., & Kaufman, J. S. (2014). Stakeholders' perspectives on community-based participatory research to enhance mental health services. *American Journal of Community Psychology, 54*(3–4), 397–408. https://doi.org/10.1007/s10464-014-9677-8

Collins, S. E., Clifasefi, S. L., Stanton, J., Straits, K. J. E., Gil-Kashiwabara, E., Rodríguez Espinosa, P., Nicasio, A. V., Andrasik, M. P., Hawes, S. M., Miller, K. A., Nelson, L. A., Orfaly, V. E., Duran, B. M., & Wallerstein, N. (2018). Community-based participatory research (CBPR): Towards equitable involvement of community in psychology research. *American Psychologist, 73*(7), 884–898. https://doi.org/10.1037/amp0000167

Committee on Assuring the Health of the Public in the 21st Century. (2003). *The future of the public's health in the 21st century*. National Academies Press.

Compton, M. T., & Shim, R. S. (2015). The social determinants of mental health. *Focus, 13*(4), 419–425. https://doi.org/10.1176/appi.focus.20150017

Corrigan, P. W., Larson, J. E., & Rüsch, N. (2009). Self-stigma and the "why try" effect: Impact on life goals and evidence-based practices. *World Psychiatry, 8*(2), 75–81. https://doi.org/10.1002/j.2051-5545.2009.tb00218.x

Corrigan, P. W., & Rao, D. (2012). On the self-stigma of mental illness: Stages, disclosure, and strategies for change. *Canadian Journal of Psychiatry, 57*(8), 464–469. https://doi.org/10.1177/070674371205700804

Crenshaw, K. (1991). Mapping the margins: Intersectionality, identity politics, and violence against women of color. *Stanford Law Review, 43*(6), 1241–1299. https://doi.org/10.2307/1229039

Dillon, E. C., Tuzzio, L., Madrid, S., Olden, H., & Greenlee, R. T. (2017). Measuring the impact of patient-engaged research: How a methods workshop identified critical outcomes of research engagement. *Journal of Patient-Centered Research and Reviews, 4*(4), 237–246. https://doi.org/10.17294/2330-0698.1458

Donabedian, A. (1988). The quality of care. How can it be assessed? *JAMA, 260*(12), 1743–1748. https://doi.org/10.1001/jama.1988.03410120089033

Driedger, S. M., Kothari, A., Morrison, J., Sawada, M., Crighton, E. J., & Graham, I. D. (2007). Using participatory design to develop (public) health decision support systems through GIS. *International Journal of Health Geographics, 6*(1), Article 53. https://doi.org/10.1186/1476-072X-6-53

Duran, B., Oetzel, J., Magarati, M., Parker, M., Zhou, C., Roubideaux, Y., Muhammad, M., Pearson, C., Belone, L., Kastelic, S. H., & Wallerstein, N. (2019). Toward health equity: A national study of promising practices in community-based participatory research. *Progress in Community Health Partnerships, 13*(4), 337–352. https://doi.org/10.1353/cpr.2019.0067

Fakhoury, W., & Priebe, S. (2007). Deinstitutionalization and reinstitutionalization: Major changes in the provision of mental healthcare. *Psychiatry, 6*(8), 313–316. https://doi.org/10.1016/j.mppsy.2007.05.008

Goodman, M. S., Thompson, V. L. S., Johnson, C. A., Gennarelli, R., Drake, B. F., Bajwa, P., Witherspoon, M., & Bowen, D. (2017). Evaluating community engagement in research: Quantitative measure development. *Journal of Community Psychology, 45*(1), 17–32. https://doi.org/10.1002/jcop.21828

Grande, S. W., Durand, M. A., Fisher, E. S., & Elwyn, G. (2014). Physicians as part of the solution? Community-based participatory research as a way to get shared decision making into practice. *Journal of General Internal Medicine, 29*(1), 219–222. https://doi.org/10.1007/s11606-013-2602-2

Guta, A., & Voronka, J. (2020). Ethical issues in community-based, participatory, and action-oriented forms of research: State of the field and future directions. In R. Iphofen (Ed.), *Handbook of research ethics and scientific integrity* (pp. 561–576). Springer.

Israel, B. A., Schulz, A. J., Parker, E. A., Becker, A. B., Allen, A. J., III, Guzman, J. R., & Lichtenstein, R. (2018). Critical issues in developing and following CBPR principles. In N. Wallerstein, B. Duran, J. Oetzel, & M. Minkler (Eds.), *Community-based participatory research for health: Advancing social and health equity* (3rd ed., pp. 31–46). Jossey-Bass.

Jagosh, J., Bush, P. L., Salsberg, J., Macaulay, A. C., Greenhalgh, T., Wong, G., Cargo, M., Green, L. W., Herbert, C. P., & Pluye, P. (2015). A realist evaluation of community-based participatory research: Partnership synergy, trust building and related ripple effects. *BMC Public Health, 15*(1), Article 725. https://doi.org/10.1186/s12889-015-1949-1

Key, K. D., Furr-Holden, D., Lewis, E. Y., Cunningham, R., Zimmerman, M. A., Johnson-Lawrence, V., & Selig, S. (2019). The continuum of community engagement in research: A roadmap for understanding and assessing progress. *Progress* in *Community Health Partnerships*, *13*(4), 427–434. https://doi.org/10.1353/cpr.2019.0064

Khodyakov, D., Stockdale, S., Jones, F., Ohito, E., Jones, A., Lizaola, E., & Mango, J. (2011). An exploration of the effect of community engagement in research on perceived outcomes of partnered mental health services projects. *Society and Mental Health*, *1*(3), 185–199. https://doi.org/10.1177/2156869311431613

Kidd, S. A., & Davidson, L. (2007). "You have to adapt because you have no other choice": The stories of strength and resilience of 208 homeless youth in New York City and Toronto. *Journal of Community Psychology*, *35*(2), 219–238. https://doi.org/10.1002/jcop.20144

Krieger, J., Allen, C., Cheadle, A., Ciske, S., Schier, J. K., Senturia, K., & Sullivan, M. (2002). Using community-based participatory research to address social determinants of health: Lessons learned from Seattle Partners for Healthy Communities. *Health Education & Behavior*, *29*(3), 361–382. https://doi.org/10.1177/109019810202900307

Lichtenstein, G., Tombari, M., Thorme, T., & Cutforth, N. (2011). Development of a national survey to assess student learning outcomes of community-based research. *Journal of Higher Education Outreach & Engagement*, *15*(2), 7–34. https://openjournals.libs.uga.edu/jheoe/article/view/839/838

Luger, T. M., Hamilton, A. B., & True, G. (2020). Measuring community-engaged research contexts, processes, and outcomes: A mapping review. *The Milbank Quarterly*, *98*(2), 493–553. https://doi.org/10.1111/1468-0009.12458

Mahone, I. H., Farrell, S. P., Hinton, I., Johnson, R., Moody, D., Rifkin, K., Moore, K., Becker, M., & Barker, M. (2011). Participatory action research in public mental health and a school of nursing: Qualitative findings from an academic–community partnership. *Journal of Participatory Medicine*, *3*, Article e-10.

Mental Health America. (n.d.). *MHA National Certified Peer Specialist*. https://mhanational.org/wp-content/uploads/2025/03/MHA-NCPS-Cert-Flyer.pdf

Minkler, M., & Wallerstein, N. (2008). *Community-based participatory research for health: From process to outcomes* (2nd ed.). Jossey-Bass.

Myrick, K., & del Vecchio, P. (2016). Peer support services in the behavioral healthcare workforce: State of the field. *Psychiatric Rehabilitation Journal*, *39*(3), 197–203. https://doi.org/10.1037/prj0000188

Nooruddin, M., Scherr, C., Friedman, P., Subrahmanyam, R., Banagan, J., Moreno, D., Sathyanarayanan, M., Nutescu, E., Jeyaram, T., Harris, M. Zhang, H. Rodriguez, A., Shaazuddin, M., Perera, M., Tuck, M., & ACCOuNT Investigators. (2020). Why African Americans say "no": A study of pharmacogenomic research participation. *Ethnicity & Disease*, *30*(Suppl. 1), 159–166. https://www.jstor.org/stable/48668434

Patient-Centered Outcomes Research Institute. (n.d.). *Engagement tool and resource repository*. https://www.pcori.org/engagement/engagement-resources/Engagement-Tool-Resource-Repository

Patient-Centered Outcomes Research Institute. (2014). *Engagement rubric for applicants*. https://www.pcori.org/sites/default/files/Engagement-Rubric.pdf

Payán, D. D., Zawadzki, M. J., & Song, A. V. (2022). Advancing community-engaged research to promote health equity: Considerations to improve the field. *Perspectives in Public Health*, *142*(3), 139–141. https://doi.org/10.1177/17579139211054118

Pelletier, J. F., Davidson, L., & Roelandt, J. L. (2009). Citizenship and recovery for everyone: A global model of public mental health. *International Journal of Mental Health Promotion, 11*(4), 45–53. https://doi.org/10.1080/14623730.2009.9721799

Rodríguez Espinosa, P., Sussman, A., Pearson, C. R., Oetzel, J. G., & Wallerstein, N. (2020). Personal outcomes in community-based participatory research partnerships: A cross-site mixed methods study. *American Journal of Community Psychology, 66*(3–4), 439–449. https://doi.org/10.1002/ajcp.12446

Sheehan, L., Ballentine, S., Agnew, L., Ali, Y., Canser, M., Connor, J., Jones, R., Laster, E., Muhammad, K., Noble, S., Smith, R., Walley, G., & Corrigan, P. W. (2016). *Inspiring change manual: A community-based participatory research manual for involving African Americans with serious mental illness in research.* Illinois Institute of Technology. https://chicagohealthdisparities.org/wp-content/uploads/2020/12/Inspiring-Change-Manual-Final_revised.pdf

Sheehan, L., Ballentine, S., Washington, L., Canser, M., Connor, J., Jones, R., Laster, E., Muhammed, K., Noble, S., Smith, R., Walley, G., Kundert, C., & Corrigan, P. (2021). Implementing community-based participatory research among African Americans with serious and persistent mental illness: A qualitative study. *Gateways: International Journal of Community Research and Engagement, 14*(1), 1–19. https://doi.org/10.5130/ijcre.v14i1.6894

Sheehan, L., Graham, A., & White, C. (2022). Using community-based participatory research to address the stigma of substance use disorder. In G. Schomerus & P. W. Corrigan (Eds.), *The stigma of substance use disorders: Explanatory models and effective interventions* (pp. 144–162). Cambridge University Press. https://doi.org/10.1017/9781108936972.008

Souleymanov, R., Kuzmanović, D., Marshall, Z., Scheim, A. I., Mikiki, M., Worthington, C., & Millson, M. (P.). (2016). The ethics of community-based research with people who use drugs: Results of a scoping review. *BMC Medical Ethics, 17*(1), Article 25. https://doi.org/10.1186/s12910-016-0108-2

Tapp, H., White, L., Steuerwald, M., & Dulin, M. (2013). Use of community-based participatory research in primary care to improve healthcare outcomes and disparities in care. *Journal of Comparative Effectiveness Research, 2*(4), 405–419. https://doi.org/10.2217/cer.13.45

Taylor, J., Namey, E., Carrington Johnson, A., & Guest, G. (2017). Beyond the page: A process review of using ethnodrama to disseminate research findings. *Journal of Health Communication, 22*(6), 532–544. https://doi.org/10.1080/10810730.2017.1317303

True, G., Alexander, L. B., & Fisher, C. B. (2017). Supporting the role of community members employed as research staff: Perspectives of community researchers working in addiction research. *Social Science & Medicine, 187*, 67–75. https://doi.org/10.1016/j.socscimed.2017.06.023

Vaughn, L. M., & Jacquez, F. (2020). Participatory research methods—Choice points in the research process. *Journal of Participatory Research Methods, 1*(1). https://doi.org/10.35844/001c.13244

Vaughn, L. M., & Lohmueller, M. (2014). Calling all stakeholders: Group-level assessment (GLA)—A qualitative and participatory method for large groups. *Evaluation Review, 38*(4), 336–355. https://doi.org/10.1177/0193841X14544903

Wallerstein, N., Oetzel, J. G., Duran, B., Magarati, M., Pearson, C., Belone, L., Davis, J., DeWindt, L., Kastelic, S., Lucero, J., Ruddock, C., Sutter, E., & Dutta, M. J. (2019). Culture-centeredness in community-based participatory research: Contributions to health education intervention research. *Health Education Research, 34*(4), 372–388. https://doi.org/10.1093/her/cyz021

Wallerstein, N. B., & Duran, B. (2006). Using community-based participatory research to address health disparities. *Health Promotion Practice, 7*(3), 312–323. https://doi.org/10.1177/1524839906289376

Index

social determinants, 79–81
social disadvantage, 75–77
sociodemographic factors, 71–75
Sociodemographic factors, 71–75
Socioeconomic status (SES), 75–76
Sociological models, of rational patients, 42–43
SODAS (situation, options, disadvantages, advantages, and solution), 105–106
Substance Abuse and Mental Health Services Administration (SAMHSA), 6–8, 107, 155–156, 172
Suicidality, 6
Summary trees, 170, 173
Support, 17–18
Support, online, 126
Supported decision making, SDM, vs., 134–144
Symptoms, as outcome measure, 180–182

T

Technology advances, 109–110
Theory of planned behavior (TPB), 41
Theory of reasoned action (TRA), 41
Thresholds (Chicago), 102, 109
TIP (Transition to Independence Process Model), 105–106
Tool development, 144
TPB (theory of planned behavior), 41
TRA (theory of reasoned action), 41
Traditional research paradigm, vs. participatory research, 194–195
Training, for participatory research, 214
Training, for SDM, 145
Transition-age youth (TAY). *See* Youth and young adults
Transition-age youth team roles, 104
Transition to adulthood, 88–93
Transition to Independence Process Model (TIP), 105–106
Trust, 11, 136
Tversky, A., 42–43
12-step models, 126

U

United Kingdom (UK), 102
University of Massachusetts Transitions to Adulthood Center for Research Young Adult Advisory Board (YAB), 102

V

Vaughn, L. M., 195, 210
Victims of crime, 76
Virtual Best Practice Guide for Youth & Young Adult Community Mental Health Providers (Thresholds), 109

W

WebMD, 173
World Health Organization (WHO), 10
World Mental Health Survey Initiative (WHO), 10
WRAP (peer-facilitated course), 137
Wraparound services, for TAY, 108

Y

YAB (University of Massachusetts Transitions to Adulthood Center for Research Young Adult Advisory Board), 102
YAYAS (Youth & Young Adult Services), 102
Youth and young adults, 87–111
development of, 94–96, 105
peer support, 106–109
and promise of SDM, 96–100
promoting SDM with, 100–110
transition to adulthood, 88–93
Youth perspectives, of SDM, 99
Youth Risk Behaviors Survey, 6
Youth & Young Adult Services (YAYAS), 102
YPS (youth/young adult peer support), 106–109

About the Editor

Patrick W. Corrigan, PsyD, is a distinguished professor of psychology at the Illinois Institute of Technology. Before that, Corrigan was a professor of psychiatry and the executive director of the University of Chicago Center for Psychiatric Rehabilitation. Corrigan has worked most of his over 30-year career providing and evaluating services for people with psychiatric disabilities with a special focus on the effect of health equity. Realizing that the benefits of psychiatric services are limited by stigma, he has spent the past 2 decades broadening his research to the prejudice and discrimination of mental illness. His work has been supported by the National Institutes of Health and the Patient-Centered Outcomes Research Institute for most of that time to, among other things, develop and lead the National Consortium on Stigma and Empowerment (https://www.stigmaandempowerment.org). This work has led to the development of the Honest, Open, Proud program (https://hopprogram.org) to erase the stigma of mental illness.

Corrigan also extended his research to mental health and social determinants (e.g., ethnicity, religion, gender identity, sexual orientation, age) and corresponding social disadvantage related to poverty, criminal justice involvement, and immigration concerns, resulting in the Chicago Health Disparities Center (https://chicagohealthdisparities.org). Corrigan has written more than 500 journal articles and 20 books. He is also editor emeritus of *Stigma and Health*, a journal of the American Psychological Association.